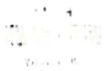

Health, Illness and Culture

Routledge Studies in Health and Social Welfare

Health, Illness and Culture

Broken Narratives

Edited by Lars-Christer Hydén
and Jens Brockmeier

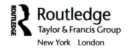

Routledge
Taylor & Francis Group
New York   London

First published 2008
by Routledge
270 Madison Ave, New York, NY 10016

Simultaneously published in the UK
by Routledge
2 Park Square, Milton Park, Abingdon, Oxon OX14 4RN

Routledge is an imprint of the Taylor & Francis Group, an informa business

© 2008 Taylor & Francis

Typeset in Sabon by IBT Global.
Printed and bound in the United States of America on acid-free paper by IBT Global.

Library of Congress Cataloging in Publication Data
  Health, illness, and culture : broken narratives / edited by Lars-Christer Hydén and
Jens Brockmeier.
    p. ; cm. — (Routledge studies in health and social welfare ; 2)
  Includes bibliographical references and index.
  ISBN-13: 978-0-415-98874-2 (hbk)
  ISBN-10: 0-415-98874-8 (hbk)
  1. Social medicine. 2. Discourse analysis, Narrative. I. Hydén, Lars-Christer, 1954–
II. Brockmeier, Jens. III. Series.
  [DNLM: 1. Attitude to Health. 2. Narration. 3. Adaptation, Psychological.
4. Culture. 5. Professional-Patient Relations. W 85 H434 2008]
  RA418.H38947 2008
  362.1—dc22
  2008001575

ISBN10: 0-415-98874-8 (hbk)
ISBN10: 0-203-89430-8 (ebk)

ISBN13: 978-0-415-98874-2 (hbk)
ISBN13: 978-0-203-89430-9 (ebk)

Contents

1 Introduction
From the Retold to the Performed Story

Lars-Christer Hydén and Jens Brockmeier

Health, Illness and Culture: Broken Narratives is a collection of studies and essays by an international group of researchers, some of whom have played a leading role in advancing the new multidisciplinary field of studies on the interrelations among, illness, disability, health, society, and culture. Since the 1980s, this field has expanded rapidly. At the same time there has been growing recognition that almost all of the phenomena within this field are mingled with processes of human meaning making, processes that typically take the form of narrative. This has added to the study of health, illness, and culture a new repertoire of forms and methods of narrative and discursive inquiry, as well as an increased degree of complexity.

Narrative itself has become the subject of an expanding but by no means homogeneous field of multidisciplinary investigation. This field, too, is marked by an expanding diversity of the theoretical approaches and methodologies brought to bear in many different areas of human communication, including everyday talk, conversational narratives, situation and genre specific discourses, fictional and nonfictional literature, and a variety of new forms of digital communication.

The overlapping and, in part, merging of these two developments has drawn attention not just to illness narratives, but also to a broad range of narrative and discursive practices that are specific to professional medical settings and, moreover, to many everyday environments of health and illness, both clinical and nonclinical. Of particular importance to all these environments, as the chapters of this book will demonstrate, are autobiographical and biographical texts and contexts. Often these contexts are only understandable within larger frameworks, such as the specific social cultures in which auto/biographical narratives are being performed.

In what follows we want to give a short overview of the field in which the study of illness and narrative overlap. Special attention will be given to tendencies, developments, and changes in the study of narrative and illness narratives, as well as on the methods and research strategies used in analyzing and interpreting illness narratives (see also Bury, 2001; Chase, 2005; Hydén, 1997; Hydén & Mishler, 1999; Mattingly, 2007). We start with reviewing research that locates illness narratives in contexts of biography, society, and culture, mainly drawing on interview studies. We then discuss studies dealing with narratives as a clinical tool and the way health care professionals use, and could use, narratives in their encounter with patients or clients. Finally, we summarize the field and relate the chapters in the current volume to ongoing currents of research and discussion, pointing to future theoretical and methodological options.

SUFFERING AND NARRATIVE

Illnesses, injuries, and disabilities are guests we never invite into our lives. Still, we all have had the experience of illness—briefly or even permanently—feeling fragile, impaired, or suffering from psychological problems due to bodily ailment or other factors. As a result, in this difficult situation we learn, whether we want to or not, about the precarious nature of what upholds and grounds our lives. Suffering from illness and trauma make us reach out toward other persons. At first most likely to partners, family members, friends, and then, if illness and suffering persists, to health care professionals—doctors, therapists, nurses, and other people with special skills and knowledge.

Reaching out means starting to talk and to tell: about the suffering, the ailments, the hurt and the changed life. In telling our stories, we hope that someone actually listens to them, listens to our experiences, and listens to our personal voices. And we trust that someone, in turn, will reach out, to treat or alleviate our suffering, or at least to recognize it. Talk and, in particular, narrative seems to be the natural way: both when we turn to other people and when we turn to ourselves as we try to come to terms with our predicament. Narrative helps us to make sense of the new life that now has to accommodate an uninvited guest. Narrative, as has often been argued, is our premier venue to give meaning to our experiences. Likewise, we order, and reflect about, events that lead or may have led up to the illness. We try to find reasons, work toward coherence (e.g., Pennebaker, 2000), find a plausible story and negotiate it, if possible and necessary, with others. We plea for hope and healing, and such pleas, too, often take the form of a story. But telling a story can also be part of our sufferings. Narrating illness and suffering is not only representing, but also expressing and performing. And it is communicating, that is, making it part of not only our own lives but also of other people.

Some illness stories are told with full voice. They are articulate and the listener is caught in a narrative web. There is an extensive literature, nonfictional as well as fictional, dealing with elaborate and often sophisticated illness stories. Often however, especially in contexts of real life and real illness, stories are not that developed. They are undecided, fragmented, broken, narrated by voices struggling to find words toward meaning and communication. These stories have been given less attention, not surprisingly perhaps. The chapters in this book are concerned with this category of illness narratives.

It seems natural that researchers in the medical and the health care professions as well as in the social sciences and the humanities have been interested in stories and storytelling about illness and suffering. Illness narratives offer a unique window on how a disease, a disability, or a trauma is lived by feeling and suffering human beings, with all its consequences for their mental, physical, and everyday life. But studying illness narratives opens up a nonreductionist, holistic perspective on how we cope with illness and suffering in still another way. It allows us to tackle questions about how, or how well, we listen to these stories as relatives and cosufferers, professionals, and researchers, and what we make of them.

ILLNESS NARRATIVE, BIOGRAPHY, AND CULTURE

Since the 1980s, research on the forms and functions of narrative in relation to illness, disability and health, as well as medicine, society, and culture, has steadily expanded. One way to look at this "narrative turn" is to view it as part of the rise of nonliterary narrative studies, a development that involved a number of different linguistic, social-scientific, psychological, philosophical, and political currents (Brockmeier & Carbaugh, 2001; Chase, 2005; Hinchman & Hinchman, 1997; Pinnegar & Daynes, 2007). Moreover, heightened multi- and inter-disciplinary awareness contributed to this growing interest in the biographical, social, and cultural contexts of human existence, both under conditions of health or sickness. From the beginning, linked to theoretical perspectives and methods sometimes called holistic, hermeneutic, and humanistic, the rise of this research domain has also coincided with changes within medicine and the health sciences, for example, the extension of research foci from acute disease towards chronic illness.

In hindsight, we might recognize as a central concern and motive of the new interest in illness narratives what Elliot Mishler (1984), in his conceptualization of the encounter between patients and medical professionals, described as the a struggle between the "voice of the life world" and the "voice of medicine." As Mishler pointed out, in a typical medical encounter the voice of the life world tends to be suppressed in favor of the voice of medicine. As a consequence, there are severe limitations to the extent of which patients can make themselves understood by articulating their own versions of their problems. But even before, researchers had been interested in how people suffering from illness are affected in their daily lives, how they define themselves, and see their illness "from the inside"—as opposed to the perspective of the medical institution (e.g., Brody, 1987; Kleinman, 1988).

As has often been pointed out, illnesses and disabilities tend to disrupt everyday life, question corresponding forms of knowledge, and challenge social relationships. In this sense, they constitute biographical threats, disrupting one's sense of continuity, identity, and autobiographical coherence (Bury, 1982; Medved & Brockmeier, 2008). The onset of illness, impairment, and suffering often raises fundamental questions about the relation of the "intruding events" to one's life, and answers are not always easily at hand. One way individuals cope is to situate the suffering within the context of their ongoing autobiographical narratives. Narrativizing experience of illness, its symptoms and interpretations, typically means situating them in a life–world context, which often overlaps with one's autobiographical context. At the same time it offers a variety of biographical perspectives, intertwining illness and diverse forms and genres of life writing (Couser, 1997, 2004.)

This is true both for oral narratives told to family members, friends, or researchers in interviews, and extended written narratives intended to be read by a larger, anonymous audience—books about the illness experience addressing other suffers. Such narrative reconstruction can provide a space that encompasses the illness event and its experience within a specific life–world, recreating in this way a new mode of interrelatedness (Charon, 2006; Frank, 1995; Kleinman, 1988; Williams, 1984). It appears that people who are ill tend to weave the threads of their illnesses and their presumed origins and therapeutic trajectories together with their personal life stories and identity constructions. What runs through all this is the quest for answers to questions as why this happened to them, what could be the "deeper" meaning of it, and what is there to hope for in the future (e.g., Charmaz, 1991; Becker, 1997; Jordens, Little, Paul, & Sayer, 2001; Smith & Sparkes, 2005; Sparkes & Smith, 2002).

This kind of research is typically interview-based. Researchers are interested in the start of the illness, its discovery, effects, diagnosis and treatment, and its further development and consequences. Often they operate with an idea of illnesses as developing along a linear temporal trajectory, with a more or less distinct start, development, and some sort of endpoint, be it recovery, chronic illness, and disability, or death. As a consequence, these interview narratives tend to follow a chronological story line. Events are represented and related to each other as they follow upon each other in a natural succession: the first not only leading to, but also causing the next event, or even a chain of events. A problem with this approach is that time is viewed as a fundamental principle of narrative and its organization, not as an option of meaning making, a resource that can be used by narrators to explore life possibilities, to play through different autobiographical strategies, to give meaning and significance to some experiences that are foregrounded, while other experiences are backgrounded or simply skipped—in short, to configure or reconfigure identity (Bülow & Hydén, 2003; Brockmeier, 2000; Ricoeur, 1991a, 1991b).

In his book *The Wounded Storyteller,* Arthur Frank (1995) has pointed out different ways in which time and temporalization have been used in telling illness narratives. He identifies three main storylines specifying relations between patients' selves, bodies, illnesses, and their expectations for the future: narratives of "restitution," "chaos," and "quest." Frank argues that these three storylines or plots can all be found in patients' illness narratives in varying degrees and in various combinations. A *restitution* narrative depicts illness as a temporary and limited impairment or affliction; the afflicted individual is positioned as the same person as before the onset, and when the illness has passed or the patient is in remission, he or she is expected to return to their former levels of functioning. On this account, then, being ill does not alter the identity of the ill person. In contrast, the *chaos* storyline represents life as radically disrupted. The self is submerged in the illness, chaos reigns, symptoms are severe and irreversible, and the future is unpredictable. The third plot model, the *quest*, articulates a sense of self that has already been changed fundamentally by the illness. Being ill initiates a journey toward new experiences and a new identity. As witnesses to their own transformation, narrators of quest stories believe they have learned something valuable that they can bring home and pass along to others, particularly to other sufferers.

The illness narratives Frank examines are told by people suffering from illnesses, often of fatal character, or by relatives of these people. These narratives are meant to be read by others in the same situation, as a way of communicating experience and knowledge that, for Frank, has no place in the world of biomedicine; in fact, it is often excluded and suppressed. They are texts that open up the sphere of everyday life and a phenomenological sense of being, sharing dimensions of the illness experience normally held at bay: the subjective world of suffering and disability, the dependence of the ill individual on others, death, and life's ultimate concerns (see also Frank, 2004). But the auto/biographical perspective not only widens the concept, as well as the experience of and reflection about, illness; it also enriches notions of everyday life and the life world.

Written and published illness narratives often conform to established literary genres and conventions, even if these commonly do not originate in the field of mostly oral illness discourse. For Ann Hawkins (1993), "pathographies" emerge from recurrent literary metaphors and myths. She argues that narrators of illness stories may make use of established narrative genres and literary conventions to reconfigure their lives and illness experiences in culturally recognisable and acceptable forms. She highlights four salient "metaphors" frequently occurring in modern American pathography: the battle, the journey, rebirth, and what she calls "healthy-mindedness." Each of these metaphors imply strategies to organize experiences of illness and treatment that create meaningful trajectories of coping.

One of Hawkins's central metaphors is based on the myth of rebirth. It shows a close parallel to what Frank dubbed the quest narrative. In both, the transformation of "self" through illness is central to the "self's rebirth": a patient who suffered a severe life crisis, over came it, and emerged regenerated as a new human being. Frequently, Hawkins claims, such narratives are organized into three parts. The first regards the time before the onset of illness, often viewed retrospectively as marked by an unhealthy life style that now is recognized and rejected. This leads in the second part to a crisis accompanying the onset of illness which, in the process, might have become a matter of life or death. This finally gives way to the third part, the actual rebirth or regeneration, the resolution of the crisis, and entry into a new life with a different appreciation of the world. The entire plot structure, Hawkins suggests, draws upon, and replaces, traditional religious conversion stories, most famously, perhaps, that of the sinner who in the moment of great despair experiences God, realizes his or her sinful life, regrets it, undergoes conversion, and begins a new God-fearing life. Hawkins shows that many narrative elements of pathographies make use of deeply rooted literary and religious resources.

Several researchers working with interview methods and ethnographic material have pointed to the wider cultural and historical embedding of the narratives told by ill and disabled people. Andrew Sparkes and Brett Smith (2002; Smith & Sparkes, 2005) have examined the identity narratives of men who suffer from spinal cord injury, demonstrating the manifold ways in which they are connected to the dominant cultural discourse about men in the United Kingdom. The individuals they interviewed were former rugby players. For these men, before the injury, their bodies were in many ways taken for granted. Being central to their never-questioned masculine self-image, their bodies were inscribed in the wider cultural discourses that maintained and affirmed hegemonic forms of masculinity, of what it means of living a life as a young man. Suffering spinal cord injuries for these men meant that their bodies "dys-appeared" and they no longer were able to tell and think about themselves as embodied masculine and athletic narratives identities. For "the narratives that have been made available in the past and are available now to these men through the world of sport are extremely problematic in terms of enabling them to construct different body–self relationships and different identities in the future" (Sparkes & Smith, 2002, pp. 280–1). The same cultural discourse that enabled these men before their injury to live the lives they considered meaningful, became the foremost obstruction after the injury in their search for a new form of life and a new narrative identity. In a comparable cultural key, Vera Skultans (2003) has explored how illness narratives of depressed patients in Latvia, a former Soviet state, are torn between traditional popular beliefs, the introduction of new psychiatric terminologies and ideas, and radical changes in everyday life brought about by the political, social, and cultural development after the end of the Communist regime in 1989.

Telling stories in interviews, as in any social context, means inviting the listener to share, contemplate, and evaluate the experiences of others. Every story, as short, vague, and fragmented it is, appeals to understanding, reaches out to someone. All narrative communication and interaction has a performative dimension. Telling a story is performing it, acting out a process of interpreting, constituting, and positioning one's experience. It is an enacting of identity. Several researchers and scholars have emphasized that all oral narrative is embodied, and to a degree also all written narrative. The embodying of one narrative reality may at the same time question another version of reality, that is, challenge *another's* version of reality. What is triggered, in this way, is a process of negotiation and reembodying.

Against this background, Kristin Langellier (2001) has analyzed an extensive narrative told by a woman who had undergone mastectomy as a result of breast cancer. Langellier demonstrates that, in illness, the body is always under threat of being colonized, not only by social stigma and cultural images of health and perfection, but also by the dominant biomedical discourse. For everyone suffering from severe illnesses, Langellier argues, it is essential to proactively define and redefine their own bodies, to recapture and reappropriate it. She shows that for this woman tattooing the scar of her mastectomy and telling a story about this is a way to regain agency, both in relation to clinical professionals as well as to herself. It is a way of enacting the right to invest her "new" body and its surgical trajectory with meaning, her own meaning. The tattoo becomes a performed identity, supported by the stories embedding the tattoo in various acts of self-definition. "The wounded storyteller," Langellier (2001) writes, "narrates a story of the body through the body" (p. 146).

CLINICAL NARRATIVES

"[The] tale of complaints becomes the text that is to be decoded by the practitioner cum diagnostician," Arthur Kleinman (1988, p. 17) wrote in his pathbreaking book, *The Illness Narratives*. Kleinman, a psychiatrist and anthropologist, was one of the first (together with Good, 1994, and Csordas, 1994) to establish what became known as the interpretive or meaning-centered paradigm of the study of illness narrative, especially in medical anthropology (see Mattingly, 2007). We already mentioned the basic assumption: For patients to tell stories about their illnesses is a way to create meaning and cope with their particular experiences. For the medical practitioner it therefore is necessary to be able to listen, understand, and interpret these narratives in order to acquire a more detailed clinical picture of the patient. In this perspective, the medical practitioner must become an expert also of the patient's narrative, both to produce a correct diagnosis and to propose an appropriate treatment (Hunter, 1991, 2005).

Kleinman, therefore, is not primarily interested in the patient's narratives as such but in the clinician listening and making sense of the patient's narrative in order to be a better clinician. In other words, the focus is on the intersubjective dynamics in the relationship between teller and listener. Medicine has a long tradition of mistrusting the voice of the patient and instead listening to "objective" signs that are the "evidence-based" results of physical exams, laboratory reports, and an ever expanding repertoire of biomedical diagnostic technologies (Armstrong, 2002). Typically, thus, medical doctors have not been not trained to listening to patients, let alone understanding and interpreting their narratives. This insight was the point of departure of the work of Rita Charon (2006; Charon & Montello, 2002) on "narrative medicine" that has proved to be influential on many new programmes in North American medical schools.

Charon has made a plea for the development of a specific "narrative medicine" that takes into account the central role of the physician absorbing, interpreting, and responding to patients' stories. She argues that it is part of the basics of clinical life that medical doctors act as narrative experts, attentively listening to and deciphering the narrative fabric of illness. To be conscious that many stories put forward existential questions also includes the awareness that there often are no clear answers to these questions. The narrative-conscious physician faces more clearly and more often than the mere biomedical practitioner the limits of their professional scope.

The role of narrative has been discovered crucial to many different therapeutic aspects of clinical work. Cheryl Mattingly (1998) has investigated how health professionals in many different fields try to shape their strategies of treatment, its course, and the process of recovery into a coherent narrative plot which she calls "therapeutic emplotment." Placed in the context of "healing dramas," physical dysfunctions and the daily tedium of routine rehabilitation may take on new meaning and thus become more endurable for the hard working professional. The form of therapeutic emplotment may also influence the patient's time horizon for the course of their illness and its treatment. In establishing a link between the medical interventions and the trajectory of recovery, it might engender hope of eventual cure (Mattingly & Garro, 2000).

Obviously, narrative is not a neutral instrument or an indifferent tool of communication in the encounter between patient and health care professional. It can be a site of struggle, not least about whose narrative is it that is being told. Who is to determine which narrative about the patient's illness will be the dominant one (Clark & Mishler, 1992; Mishler, 2005)? Many studies have shown that in typical clinical encounters physicians either ignore or interrupt patients' accounts, and they do so all the more the more these accounts are formulated in narrative form. But there *is*, of course, narrative in the traditional clinical business. The usual story put forward by the doctor has the form of a chronicle in which signs and symptoms are ordered sequentially but removed from the larger context of patients' lives. What also is removed are the meanings patients give to their illnesses, the symptoms and the personal phenomenology of their illness experiences and the way the illness impacts on their everyday life, individually and socially. To become able and sensitive enough to perceive these contextualised stories, physicians must relinquish, or at least moderate, their institutional dominance and their role as the sole and authoritarian expert of matters of health and illness, of imposing "their" biomedical plot of illness and cure; instead, they have to move toward what Charon (2006) describes as becoming attentive, responsive, and responsible listeners. And what's more, they have to encourage patients to tell their stories, which often are quiet and broken, and indeed hard to recognize as stories at all (Medved & Brockmeier, 2004).

PROTOTYPE CASES OF ILLNESS NARRATIVES

The field of illness narratives is all but a well-marked academic or clinical terrain, not to mention that it also extends into a literary terrain (see, e.g., the 25 volumes of the Journal *Literature and Medicine,* presently [2007/2008] edited by Maura Spiegel and Rita Charon)—a terrain which our book, however, does not cover. Not surprisingly there are many different views and approaches to what narrative is and how it is supposed to be examined. One way of thinking about the variety of definitions of narrative in general and illness narrative in particular is that different researchers, working in a wide spectrum of culturally diverse practical and theoretical environments, start from different prototypical cases of narratives. The cognitive psychologist Elenor Rosch (1978) once suggested that much of our categorical thinking is structured around the best example of something. In what follows, other instances are grouped around this prototypical case, forming what we might call phenomenological family resemblance, to borrow Wittgenstein's term. Let us illustrate this idea by referring to four important prototypical examples in the field of illness narrative, each outlining a particular concept of narrative and a way how it is best approached.

The first prototype idea is narrative as a *retelling* of stories already told by someone else. An elemental example of this is the physician retelling a story the patient told them before. Consider classical case studies like those by Sigmund Freud, Alexander Luria, or Oliver Sacks. In more recent variants, the focus has shifted from the patient's stories to the doctor's own experience and its narrative underpinnings (e.g., Borkan, Reis, Steinmatz, & Medalie, 1999; Greenhalgh & Hurwitz, 1998; Hurwitz, Greenhalgh & Skultons, 2004). In these "retellings" of illness narratives we do not hear the voice of the patient but the voice of the doctor and his or her medical emplotment.

A second protoypical narrative is the *interview narrative*. This is primarily produced by social scientists and psychologists interested in the subjective illness experience against a psychological, social, and cultural background. The focus here is on narratives told by patients/clients and, in some cases, relatives. Most of this research is based on small samples of patient interviews and the questions raised deal with, for example, whose voices and perspectives are represented in an illness narrative (e.g., Little et al., 2002).

The third prototypical case highlights the *coconstruction* of stories: the way stories are jointly produced in the interaction between interviewer and interviewee, medical doctors and patient, psychoanalyst and analysant. This idea is well expressed by psychoanalyst Roy Schafer's (1992) "relationalist approach." For Schafer, the psychoanalytic encounter is the place in which a joint narrative is being negotiated, a discursive forum with "two subjectivities meeting in a unique situation and creating a third space in which new experience becomes possible" (Schafer, 2004, p. 250). This approach brings together a number of tendencies exploring narrative intersubjectivity that also include the humanities. Already in 1977, literary theorist Mary Louise Pratt wrote that in telling a story, the teller is "inviting his addressees to join him in contemplating it, evaluating it, and responding to it" (Pratt, 1977, p. 135).

Finally, there is the prototype of a *performed narrative*, or of *narrative as performance*. In the wake of speech act theory, Goffman's (1973, 1981) studies of human's expressive social behavior, and Judith Butler's (e.g., 1990) explorations of gender performativity, many researchers of "everyday narratives," including illness narratives, have come to view storytelling in a key of performative action (e.g., Langellier & Peterson, 2004). To understand storytelling as performing means imagining the space between teller and listener being filled in a physical, spatial, and bodily fashion. In telling, the entire bodily presence and identity of the narrator are staged, inviting the listener and conarrator to join the performance in a similar enactive mode. Conceiving of narrative as a performative mode seems to be a particularly promising approach in order to understand forms of communication and reflection in individuals suffering from severe illnesses and disabilities.

BROKEN NARRATIVES: THE BOOK

The authors of this volume have different backgrounds in psychology, sociology, anthropology and ethnography, philosophy, social work, and the health care professions. But more than their disciplinary (and often multidisciplinary) and professional (and multiprofessional) backgrounds, they represent a common research interest in forms and aspects of what we have called *broken narratives*. By that we do not want to stake a claim or offer a precise descriptive or normative label; rather we conceive of broken narrative as an open and fluid concept, emphasizing problematic, precarious, and damaged narratives told by people who in one way or another have trouble telling their stories, be it due to injury, disability, dementia, pain, grief, psychological or neurological trauma. The collection of essays of this volume presents both a number of theoretical and methodological approaches to the narrative field of health, illness, and culture, and various views of the complexity of the narratives produced in this field.

In his chapter, "Language, Experience, and the 'Traumatic Gap': How to Talk About 9/11?," Jens Brockmeier poses the question whether there is a language to capture, and cope with, the experience of trauma. Examining eyewitness accounts of the catastrophe of 9/11 in Manhattan, his essay explores the registers of language (and the appropriateness of questionnaires and interview formats) in articulating such extreme existential experiences.

In the next chapter, "Broken and Vicarious Voices in Narratives," Lars-Christer Hydén discusses different strategies used by people who suffer from communicative disorders and disabilities. The focus is on persons with brain trauma and dementia and the way medical staff and family members help them to talk about their experiences. When a person lacks the ability to articulate himself or herself, to have an own voice, it is not just the sounds that are missing but also the ability to form stories. When another person has to serve as a vicarious voice, they not only loan out their sounding voice, but also to act as an organizing voice trying to figure out which story to tell.

Maria Medved and Jens Brockmeier, in their chapter "Talking About the Unthinkable: Neurotrauma and the 'Catastrophic Reaction,'" examine the narratives of a woman with brain injury, but from a point of view different from Hydén's chapter. Medved and Brockmeier discuss how the study of narratives, as fragmented as they may be, can help us understand the dynamics involved in an overwhelming psychological reaction to brain damage. How do people whose cognitive and linguistic capacities are seriously affected by neurotrauma try to make sense out of what has happened to them? In their analysis the authors combine a neuropsychological view that draws on ideas of neurologist Kurt Goldstein with a narrative-analytical view, pointing out similarities and differences.

Narratives and the telling of narratives are often thought of as having a "healing power." Cheryl Mattingly examines this question in her chapter "Stories That are Ready to Break." Mattingly understands narrative in the course of clinical care neither as something that heals, nor as something that obstructs healing, but rather as a fragile act that, even when it seems to be most promising as an instrument for healing, can easily fail and be abandoned.

In Chapter 6, "Globally Distributed Silences, and Broken Narratives About HIV," Georg Drakos asks in what ways does silence about HIV shape the very conditions of living with HIV and, eventually, dying of AIDS. Narratives, Drakos argues, can constitute one kind of reality and simultaneously silence another, a double bind that characterizes the lives of many individuals living with HIV, turning their stories into ongoing negotiation about what reality is.

In his chapter, "Caring for the Dead: Broken Narratives of Internment," Arthur Frank is concerned with a similar problem: with stories that "resist telling." The narratives in Frank's study are broken because, as he argues, it is the nature of the teller's experiences that his experiences do not and cannot coalesce into a cohesive whole. On the other hand, it is this "whole-ness" that in an entire tradition of narrative studies, as well as illness nar-rative studies, has been evoked. Frank shows that the storyteller struggles between a need to let the story act as a form of what grief counselors call *closure* and, opposed to that, a sense that any story presenting the experi-ence as complete and completed would betray what happened.

In Chapter 8, "'You Have to Ask a Little': Troublesome Storytelling About Contested Illness," Pia Bülow presents an analysis of interviews with a man suffering from a contested illness, chronic fatigue syndrome (CFS). She shows that the stories of this man, while they appear at first sight as broken narratives, are attempts to articulate experiences previously untold; they are stories in progress. This leads to the question of what makes sto-ries about contested illnesses "true" illness narratives. And how do doubt and scepticism toward one's narratives influence their telling in medical encounters as well as in everyday life?

In Chapter 9, "Break-Up Narratives," Margareta Hydén explores the sto-ries women have told her after leaving their abusive men. These break-up nar-ratives play an important role in determining along what lines her (re)formed life trajectories might develop. A break-up from a violent marriage is generally conceived of as a single event, composing the demarcation line between "the past evil and the future good life." In emphasizing the relief and joy, and cel-ebrating the new opportunities that often come along with a break-up, this version of a break-up experience does, however, not leave much space for the agony and pain that also come with it. In fact, as Margareta Hydén demon-strates, the stories of women are not told along these lines but rather reflect a multiplicity of feelings. Time is not linear in these stories. The battered wom-an's break-up narrative does not have a finite ending, a point at which con-tinuation is unthinkable and at which all loose ends are tied up. They reflect a world in which the future is open, admitting the presence of possibilities that could add desirable as well as undesirable parts to the woman's past.

Finally in Chapter 10, "Beyond Narrative: Dementia's Tragic Promise," Mark Freeman deals with the limits of narrative understanding. Freeman's point of departure is an autobiographical one: His mother has been afflicted by Alzheimer's disease. Struggling to understand her condition and increas-ingly disorganized attempts to live a life on her own, Freeman offers a series of fundamental thoughts upon the way people may be more tied to concrete situations in the here and now than to a life narrative which, after all, is based on a process of abstraction and self-reflection.

REFERENCES

Armstrong, D. (2002). *A new history of identity: A sociology of medical knowl-edge*. London: Palgrave.

Becker, G. (1997). *Disrupted lives: How people create meaning in a chaotic world.* Berkeley, CA: University of California Press.

Borkan, J., Reis, S., Steinmatz, D., & Medalie, J. H. (Eds.). (1999). *Patients and doctors. Life-changing stories from primary care.* Madison, WI: The University of Wisconsin Press.

Brockmeier, J. (2000). Autobiographical time. *Narrative Inquiry, 10,* 51–73.

Brockmeier, J., & Carbaugh, D. (2001). Introduction. In J. Brockmeier & D. Carbaugh (Eds.), *Narrative and identity: Studies in autobiography, self and culture* (pp. 1–22). Amsterdam & Philadelphia: John Benjamins.

Brody, H. (1987). *Stories of sickness.* New Haven, CT: Yale University Press.

Bülow, P., & Hydén, L. C. (2003). In dialogue with time: Identity and illness in narratives about chronic fatigue. *Narrative Inquiry, 13,* 71–97.

Bury, M. (1982). Chronic illness as biographical disruption. *Sociology of Health and Illness, 4,* 167–182.

Bury, M. (2001). Illness narratives: Fact or fiction. *Sociology of Health & Illness, 23,* 263–285.

Butler, J. (1990). *Gender trouble: Feminism and the subversion of identity.* New York & London: Routledge.

Charmaz, K. (1991). *Good days, bad days. The self in chronic illness and time.* New Brunswick, NJ: Rutgers University Press.

Charon, R. (2006). *Narrative medicine: Honoring the stories of illness.* New York: Oxford University Press.

Charon, R., & Montello, M. (2002). *Stories matter: The role of narrative in medical ethics.* New York: Routledge.

Chase, S. E. (2005). Narrative inquiry. In N. Denzin & Y. S. Lincoln (Eds.), *The Sage handbook of qualitative research,* (3rd ed., pp. 651–679). Thousand Oaks, CA: Sage.

Clark, J. A., & Mishler, E. G. (1992). Attending to patients' stories: Reframing the clinical task. *Sociology of Health and Illness, 14,* 344–371.

Couser, G. T. (1997). *Recovering bodies: Illness, disability, and life writing.* Madison, WI: The University of Wisconsin Press.

Couser, G. T. (2004). *Vulnerable subjects: Ethics and life writing.* Ithaca, NY: Cornell University Press.

Csordas, T. (Ed.). (1994). *Embodiment and experience: The existential ground of culture and self.* Cambridge, MA: Harvard University Press.

Frank, A. W. (1995). *The wounded storyteller: Body, illness, and ethics.* Chicago: The University of Chicago Press.

Frank, A. W. (2004). *The renewal of generosity: Illness, medicine, and how to live.* Chicago: The University of Chicago Press.

Goffman, E. (1973). *The presentation of self in everyday life.* Woodstock, NY: Overlook Press.

Goffman, E. (1981). *Forms of talk.* Philadelphia: University of Pennsylvania

Good, B. (1994). *Medicine, rationality, and experience: An anthropological experience.* New York: Cambridge University Press.

Greenhalgh, T., & Hurwitz, B. (Eds.). (1998). *Narrative based medicine: Dialogue and discourse in clinical practice.* London: BMJ Books.

Hawkins, A. H. (1993). *Reconstructing illness. Studies in pathography.* West Lafayette: Purdue University Press.

Hinchman, L. P., & Hinchman, S. K. (Eds.). (1997). *Memory, identity, community: The idea of narrative in the human sciences.* Albany, NY: State University of New York Press.

Hunter, K. M. (1991). *Doctor's stories: The narrative structure of medical knowledge.* Princeton, NJ: Princeton University Press.

Hunter, K. M. (2005). *How doctors think: Clinical judgment and the practice of medicine.* Oxford: Oxford University Press.

Hurwitz, B., Greenhalgh, T., & Skultans, V. (Eds.). (2004). *Narrative research in health and illness.* Oxford: Blackwell Publishing.

Hydén, L. C. (1997). Illness and narrative. *Sociology of Health and Illness, 19,* 48–69.

Hydén, L. C., & Mishler, E. G. (1999). Medicine and language. *Annual Review of Applied Lingustics, 19,* 174–192.

Jordens, C. F. C., Little, M., Paul, K., & Sayer, E.-J. (2001). Life disruption and generic complexity: A social linguistic analysis of narratives of cancer illness. *Social Science and Medicine, 53,* 1227–1236.

Kleinman, A. (1988). *The illness narratives: Suffering, healing, and the human condition.* New York: Basic Books.

Langellier, K. (2001). "You're marked": Breast cancer, tattoo, and the narrative performance of identity. In J. Brockmeier & D. Carbaugh (Eds.), *Narrative and identity: Studies in autobiography, self and culture* (pp. 145–184). Amsterdam & Philadelphia: John Benjamins.

Langellier, K., & Peterson, E. E. (2004). *Storytelling in daily life: Performing narrative.* Philadelphia: Temple University Press.

Little, M., Jordens, C. F. C., Paul, K., Sayer, E.-J., Cruickshank, J. A., Stegeman, J., et al. (2002). Discourse in different voices: reconciling N = 1 and N=many. *Social Science and Medicine, 55,* 1079–1087.

Mattingly, C. (1998). *Healing dramas and clinical plots: The narrative structure of experience.* New York: Cambridge University Press.

Mattingly, C. (2007). Acted narratives: From storytelling to emergent dramas. In D. J. Clandinin (Ed.), *Handbook of narrative inquiry: Mapping a methodology* (pp. 405–425). Thousand Oaks, CA: Sage.

Mattingly, C., & Garro, L. C. (Eds.). (2000). *Narrative and the cultural construction of illness and healing.* Berkeley, CA: University of California Press.

Medved, M. I., & Brockmeier, J. (2004). Making sense of traumatic experiences: Telling your life with Fragile X syndrome. *Qualitative Health Research, 14,* 741–759.

Medved, M. I., & Brockmeier, J. (2008). Continuity amid chaos: Neurotrauma, loss of memory, and sense of self. *Qualitative Health Research, 18,* 469–479.

Mishler, E. G. (1984). *The discourse of medicine: Dialectics of medical interviews.* Norwood, NJ: Ablex Publishing Company.

Mishler, E. G. (2005). Patient stories, narratives of resistance and the ethics of humane care: la recherche du temps perdu. *Health, 9,* 431–451.

Pennebaker, J. W. (2000). Telling stories: The health benefits of narrative. *Literature and Medicine, 19,* 3–18.

Pinnegar, S., & Daynes, J. G. (2007). Locating narrative inquiry historically: Thematics in the turn to narrative. In N. Denzin & Y. S. Lincoln (Eds.), *The Sage handbook of qualitative research* (3rd ed., pp. 3–34). Thousand Oaks, CA: Sage.

Pratt, M. L. (1977). *Toward a speech act theory of literary discourse.* Bloomington: Indiana University Press.

Rosch, E. (1978). Principles of categorization. In E. Rosch & B. B. Lloyd (Eds.), *Cognition and categorization* (pp. 27–48). New York: Lawrence Erlbaum.

Ricoeur, P. (1991a). *Narrative and time* (Vol. 3). Chicago, IL: University of Chicago Press.

Ricoeur, P. (1991b). Life in quest of narrative. In D. Wood (Ed.), *On Paul Ricoeur: Narrative and interpretation* (pp. 20–33). London: Routledge.

Schafer, R. (1992). *Retelling a life: Narration and dialogue in psychoanalysis.* New York: Basic Books.

Schafer, R. (2004). Narrating, attending, and empathizing. *Literature and Medicine, 23,* 241–251.

Skultans, V. (2003). From damaged nerves to masked depression: Inevitability and hope in Latvian psychiatric narratives. *Social Science & Medicine, 56,* 2421–2431.

Smith, B., & Sparkes, A. C. (2005). Men, sport, spinal cord injury, and narratives of hope. *Social Science and Medicine, 61,* 1095–1105.

Sparkes, A. C., & Smith, B. (2002). Sport, spinal cord injury, embodied masculinities, and the dilemmas of narrative identity. *Men and Masculinities, 4,* 258–285.

Williams, G. (1984). The genesis of chronic illness: Narrative re-construction. *Sociology of Health and Illness, 6,* 175–200.

2 Language, Experience, and the "Traumatic Gap"
How to Talk About 9/11?

Jens Brockmeier

There are many ways to tackle the relationship between language and experience. One is to listen to people who have had experiences they feel escape their words and, often enough, escape words at all. There is of course an odd paradox about listening to people in order to understand experiences that seem to evade words. This essay is about this paradox. It is concerned with such elusive experiences and how people talk about them. It draws on accounts made by eyewitnesses of the events of September 11, 2001 in Manhattan. I should say right at the beginning that my work on these accounts has been more difficult than usual. The accounts were collected as part of a larger psychological study carried out by the New York-based "National 9/11 Memory Consortium." I had been invited to study this collection of material but since the day I agreed I have felt ambivalent about the entire project; and what's more, I also have felt ambivalent about my own role in "doing research" on the reactions, reflections, and emotions of people who were immediately affected by the attacks on the World Trade Center. But let me start with how it all began.

We arrived in New York shortly after the September 2001 events. My wife and I were to take on appointments at an university in Manhattan and arrangements had been made long before. Being well aware of the city's notoriously desperate housing market, we thought ourselves to be happy when friends helped us find an apartment in a Lower Manhattan neighborhood that would have been far beyond our financial reach a few months earlier. But as 1 West Street was not only just a stone throw away from the waters of New York Harbor but also from the place where the former Twin Towers stood, many people had left the area and the rents had dropped. Just after we were settled in our new place the wind shifted, and there was this offensive smell from Ground Zero that would go on for months. The smell was produced by smoldering mountains of rubble with thousands of miles of electric cables that even months-long efforts of firefighters had not managed to put out. But "the rubble" also consisted of the remains of almost 3,000 human beings.

This fused with another ambivalence. In those days, the air in New York was not only filled with stories of death, life, and narrow escapes, but it was also the time in which public life all over America became dominated by an unparalleled wave of patriotism. Nationalism was the term used outside of the country. As we know by now, the events of 9/11 were very quickly politically "colonialized," as the *New York Times* put it, by the U.S. administration for their own agenda, with the attacks as a rationale and justification for two wars and tens of thousands more victims. It was a time, when President George W. Bush stated: You are either with us or against us.

It was a time when, listening to all kinds of haunting stories, I felt increasingly nervous as I searched for a foothold in a city that was to be my home for some years to come. Knowing this tension in my shoulders and pressure in my forehead was not only due to the special nervousness that accompanied living in the city even before the attacks, I was struggling to make up my mind in the face of a series of questions, such as how and with whom was I going to do my work, and more importantly, why I was doing it.

My work is concerned with how people make meaning of their lives. I try to understand how we make sense of our experiences, including extreme experiences, and what role narrative plays in all of this. But how can you work, "do research" on extreme experiences like suffering and trauma when exactly this suffering and trauma is being instrumentalized for what you believe is a pretext for more suffering and trauma? Is there a vocabulary, a style, a genre to articulate the tension between what the smell of dead bodies means to you as a human being and how you feel about the political claims and actions that attempt to justify themselves by referring to those same bodies?

And finally an old problem resurfaced through all this: Is there a language at all to talk about such experiences and feelings? How are we to understand the border zone between experiences we can articulate, communicate, and narrate, and those experiences we believe we cannot articulate and that seem to remain ineffable? This is a problem I, and not only I, have been struggling with for a quite a while (e.g., Brockmeier, 2002, in press; Medved & Brockmeier, 2004), a problem that I saw at the time, and still see, as being closely intertwined with the issues at stake.

But then, in one of those undecided days in which I especially felt as a struggling outsider, an anthropologist in an opaque cultural field, I found support from where I least expected it. When I, in all my all reluctance, eventually took a look at the eyewitness accounts I was immediately drawn into them. Apparently many of those who were directly affected by the events of September 11 were troubled by the very same questions. In fact, many seemed to have been confronted with strikingly similar ambivalences, both in terms of the nature of their experiences and their effability, and in terms of the intermingling of the individual and private with the political and historical.

In more technical terms, what most eyewitnesses had experienced was serious trauma, and in their accounts they struggled to come to terms with this experience and the resulting consequences. At the same time, many of them were realizing the larger political implications of the events and the pending military reactions of the U.S. government. Now, "struggling to come to terms with experience" is, again, not very technical ("trauma technical") language. But then, again, is there any technical language to come to terms with such an extreme experience?

Before I tackle the question of whether language can speak about the landscape of experience we have come to label "trauma," I want to say a few more words about the research project whose material I eventually came to use for my own investigation.[1] After all, this was a type of research, so common in academic psychology, that made me feel even more entangled among conflicting agendas. The project was carried out by a group of leading psychologists from 12 American universities (including Harvard, Yale, Stanford, Columbia, New York University, and The New School) who were responsible for setting up "The National 9/11 Memory Consortium." Using the same approach as traditional *flashbulb* memory studies, the researchers began, right after September 11, to investigate the kinds of memories people in the United States as well as abroad currently had, and would have in the future, of the events and of themselves experiencing them.[2] The basis of the "The 9/11 National Memory Survey on the Terrorist Attacks" was a questionnaire of roughly 40 mainly short answer questions and rating scales. The questionnaire was distributed 4 days after the attacks and answered by 1,495 participants in the United States and in Europe, 546 of them residents of New York City.

At the end of the questionnaire some additional questions were included, inviting participants to describe what the events of September 11 meant to them personally, to the city of New York, and to the United States in general. Although participants were explicitly asked in the questionnaire to answer only "in a brief paragraph," they sometimes went to great lengths providing what might be called a narrative surplus. To be sure, this narrative surplus was unexpected and presumably unintended by the lead researchers who designed the study. Now, my interest of course focussed on this narrative surplus, these open-ended comments and personal remarks. Although I came to see myself living in that city more like a cultural anthropologist—or an investigative journalist, for that matter—who examines all available kinds of material, bits and pieces of human experience in order to make sense of what is going on in the lives and minds of people, in this essay I draw primarily on the accounts of 26 eyewitnesses, people who were, at the time of the catastrophe, at or near the Twin Towers in Lower Manhattan. These are the reports of individuals who, as one of them put it, had it happen "in their faces." Hand-written and on average one page in length, they reflect the experience of that morning a few days later, putting them in a personal and often autobiographical context. They include thoughts, intentions, and anxieties regarding their own future, and—on a more fundamental moral and existential plane—thoughts about the meaning and significance of their lives. They also include reflections about how to talk about an experience that, as several medical studies have reported, led many people to long-standing symptoms of posttraumatic stress disorder. In the words of a 45-year-old woman who saw the first plane crashing above her into the North Tower, commenting on what it means to her:

> It means, [since then] I have had constant stomach aches. It means every time I hear a plane or helicopter above, my pulse shoots up. It means crying for a few minutes several times every day since the attack. . .

THE GAP BETWEEN EXPERIENCE AND WORDS

It has often been noted that there is a gap between how one experiences trauma and how one communicates such an experience. Those who report a traumatic experience often feel that their accounts do not adequately or satisfactorily capture such experience, if it can be adequately and satisfactorily articulated at all. Where does this gap come from? There are a number of answers to this question, each drawing on different views of the relationship between language and experience—which must not be mistaken for the relationship between language and thought. One answer emphasizes the restricted access to language in the individual who experiences a trauma. A second explanation points out the limited scope of language in general, when compared to the reach of human perception and experience and, moreover, the whole of our conscious and unconscious mental and emotional life. Lastly, the third explanation highlights the independence of emotions from language, with trauma seen primarily as an emotional experience.

I want to offer three observations that neither directly confirm or dispute any of these hypotheses, but may nevertheless help us to better understand what the traumatic gap is about, how people are aware of it, and how they attempt to bridge or narrow the gap. My observations bring to the fore different aspects of how language and experience intermingle and, by doing so, suggest a way in which to view this relationship beyond any representational notion of language. The representational notion of the relationship between language and experience conceives of language as something that expresses, reflects, or otherwise represents experience. Although this view has often been repudiated and deconstructed (by theorists as different as Wittgenstein, Heidegger, Davidson, and Derrida), many debates in psychology and psychiatry, especially in trauma theory and therapy, continue to draw on the representational assumption.

In reading the eyewitness accounts, the first observation that stands out is that there is indeed an odd inadequacy of the language used to describe both the events and their meanings in personal and emotional terms. Let me explain this by taking a closer look at the language of "singularity" and "uniqueness" by which many tried to capture their experience of that September morning. Irrespective of any political and historical point of view, what happened on that day in New York City was an absolutely exceptional experience for all those who had witnessed it. It did not come close to anything they had ever experienced in their lives. In emphasizing this dimension of singularity, uniqueness, and exceptionality, many, in hindsight, referred not only to their individual experiences but also to a historical feeling, a lost sense of safety and certainty.

A 29-year-old man, who labeled himself as a second-generation New Yorker, put it this way: "[I am] confused about my perspective of the city, country, what life will mean and be like now that we are truly not safe from attack, i.e., my paradigm has shifted to the unknown, undefined." A woman of 45 who was in her apartment near the World Trade Center when she heard "an unbelievably loud plane go by," remarked: "I no longer feel like no one can touch me just because I live in NYC." Similarly, a 62-year-old who grew up in the city stated, "Although there was some sense in the cold war that we were vulnerable, it never really hit home. Wars, as terrible as they were, occurred in Korea and Vietnam. The 'loss of American innocence' is a hackneyed phrase, but I do think we've lost a sense of invulnerability." Again, with a different accent, a 33-year-old woman from Brooklyn stated: "People [here] have lost some of the arrogance and invincibility they've always felt."

Much has been said and written about the fact that, from the very beginning, the attacks and their perception were mingled with media coverage. For most people the events and the manifold and idiosyncratic ways in which they were experienced became indistinguishable from media representations. But it was not only the nonstop live imagery and the on-the-spot reporting that framed and structured individual perception. Most people's perceiving, thinking, and imagining is influenced not just by single media events but by entire media traditions: iconographic genealogies of photographs, films, and other imagery, which are usually fused together with various narrative registers, all of which have been built up long before. It is also for this reason that a real catastrophe that is experienced in real life "will often seem eerily like its representation," as Susan Sontag (2003, p. 19) notes in her book *Regarding the Pain of Others*. As a case in point Sontag refers to the attack on the World Trade Center which "was described as 'unreal,' 'surreal,' 'like a movie,' in many of the first accounts of those who escaped from the towers or watched from nearby." She goes on to note, "[a]fter four decades of big-budget Hollywood disaster films, 'It felt like a movie' seems to have displaced the way survivors of a catastrophe used to express the short-term unassimilability of what they had gone through: 'It felt like a dream.'" Only months before the attacks on the World Trade Center and the Pentagon, the film *Pearl Harbor* was released, a costly Hollywood production which was "addicted to explosions," as film historian David Thomson (2006) writes. "As such," Thomson continues, "it was part of a climate of disaster/horror/spectacle movies so embedded on the morning of 9/11 that it's understandable if some children taking in the destruction of the Twin Towers with their Cream of Wheat asked their parents, 'Which movie is this from?'"

In one of the accounts of the 9/11 memory study, a 34-year-old man described it this way:

> I was riding my bike down 5th Avenue route to work & heard a plane flying low overhead . . . Pulled off the street and watched as the first plane banked right + crashed into tower . . . I had seen it clearly but still couldn't believe it . . . [I thought] it was sure sort of stunt, a special effect. . . .

Sontag and Thomson take up an argument that has also been brought forward by cultural theorists like Walter Benjamin and Theodor W. Adorno. Benjamin and Adorno pointed out that modern communication and culture technologies have come at a price, the "loss" of individual and authentic experience and memory. Undoubtedly, there is much evidence for this claim. On the other hand, one might wonder if modern media coverage could not also be viewed, among other things, as offering additional discursive and imaginative resources. Don't we see, hear, learn more of singular and unique events as they are covered, reported about, and magnified by the press than ever before in the history of reported witnessing? This point granted, it does not change the fact that there remains a peculiar contradiction, a clash between experience and language—including the language used by the media. This clash might be even more drastic than before because it is being enhanced and magnified by the media which, regardless of its form, employs and relies on language.

The clash, as we saw, results from a mismatch between the extraordinary extent, the sheer enormity of the events, and the altogether quite ordinary language in which they were couched. While hijacking, and the crashing of the airplanes filled with passengers into two of the biggest office towers in the world, and the subsequent collapse and pulverization of these towers, and the death of thousands of more people as a result, is a scenario of utmost monstrosity, the language used to describe it is all but singular and unique. The language is well known and all too familiar, and this is exactly the problem. The more everyday the language, the more familiar it sounds, the more it loses the horror of what it attempts to capture.

To be sure, it hardly comes as a surprise to find in the eyewitness accounts frequent use of nouns such as:

> confusion, shock, anxiety, frustration, fear, uncertainty, powerlessness, hate, helplessness, and no peace of mind.

Similarly familiar is the range of adjectives, such as:

unbelievable, incredible, impossible, terrified, scared, worried, frightened, panicked, angry, sad, vulnerable, helpless, paralyzed with fear, and depressed.

If we look at these terms from a sociolinguistic perspective, we find that the same vocabulary is typically used to describe, say, a car accident, a medical diagnosis, or a forest fire. This point is not intended to devalue everyday language use against the backdrop of other attempts to linguistically capture extreme traumatic experiences, attempts some might consider to be stylistically or aesthetically more advanced. One could, for example, think of Virginia Woolf writing about the trauma of Septimus Smith, a shell-shocked victim of the Great War; or Primo Levi and Paul Celan witnessing the Holocaust; or Homer describing the horrors experienced by Odysseus—after all, the Greek warrior was an eyewitness of the mass slaughter of Troy.

It is, however, not my intention to ponder whether there are literary forms that might be better suited for bridging the traumatic gap between experience and language, or even whether they make us more aware of this gap, by perhaps further radicalizing it, as, for example, Derrida (2005) has argued in his reading of Celan. The point I want to make here is that not only were writers and poets like Virginia Woolf, Primo Levi, Paul Celan, and Homer aware of the tension between words and extreme experiences, but also many of the eyewitnesses of September 11.

It seems that it was precisely this experience of a mismatch, the sense of a discrepancy between the personal meaning of the events and the words at hand, that many participants were grappling with. After being asked what the attack meant to him, a 25-year-old New Yorker stated: "It means a lot of things to me which I can't put into words." When asked the same question, a 39-year-old Latino man who spent all his life in the city said: "I feel that my mourning is not enough to portray my feelings." A woman of 36 who was at Liberty Plaza, across the road from the South Tower, when the first plane exploded, wrote about the personal meaning of the events: "I don't think I can really comprehend the significance of the attack to me. Had things happened in a different sequence I could have been injured or killed but I really haven't internalized this."

After having read comments like these, I believed to recognize in them the same kind of uncertainty and ambivalence I had experienced in myself, even though I found it here in an incommensurably more overwhelming and, indeed, existential context of experience. What I did *not* find (apart from two exceptions) was the language of patriotism, nationalism, and revenge used by the political class and the media in those days.

For many it seemed difficult to distinguish between the personal meaning of the attack (asked for in the questionnaire) and its larger political and historical meanings. But then, is this really surprising? Experiencing an event like this, how can one tell the private from the public, the personal from the political? "The historical" literally invaded "the private." This is what a woman of 31 from Brooklyn had to say:

> I didn't go home Tuesday night (was too freaked out to ride the subway to Brooklyn). I didn't accomplish much work on Tuesday, Thursday, or Friday, and our work schedule was thrown off. Building was closed on Wednesday . . . Services were cut off . . . Also, I've stopped writing my morning journal pages . . .

A 53-year-old woman who was walking near the towers when the first plane exploded said:

> Whenever I hear an airplane, I get tense. I am using the wrong keys for my door . . . Have nightmares and my alpha stage before sleep has very discombobulating thoughts. I am petrified, tired + not myself. I feel like I have been through a twilight zone episode. *Masks Military Police State Troopers Scary.*

And a 72-year-old academic from an university in Greenwich Village, who went eight times to give blood on the day after the attack, said this about his emotions (which he added to the six emotions—sad, angry, fear, confusion, frustration, shock—given in the questionnaire and which were to be rated on a scale):

> Intense feelings of regret for the ways US has behaved in the world which helped provoke the attack. A sense of guilt for not doing more to help build positive relationships among people. Deep feeling of closeness and caring for family members & solidarity with those with losses.

METAPHORS AND IMAGES OF THE EXTREME

A second observation is that the felt gap between the traumatic experience and words is only half the story. There also are attempts to bridge or, at least, narrow the gap. One option is to extend the semantic resources of the vocabulary (nouns, adjectives, and verbs—the common currency of a language) by using figurative speech. Often metaphors and images are more sensitive and expressive, and therefore are preferred in talk about unusual, multilayered, and contradictory phenomena. Furthermore, they draw attention and affect to speakers and what they have to say. By breaking with routinized ways of talking and imagining, metaphors not only invite different ways of perceiving and thinking, but they also suggest relationships that one did not see before. They not only just represent or reflect reality, but they also create novel realties. Indeed, new or vital metaphors permit us to see aspects of the world that they themselves help constitute.

One of the questions in the questionnaire was whether the attack "inconvenienced daily activities," and one young woman replied: "I wouldn't call it an inconvenience. . . . My whole idea of daily routine was blasted." This metaphor literally transfers the physical scenario into one's everyday life, both practical and mental. In as far as it uses a central element of the catastrophe (the blast), to characterize something completely different (a change in one's idea of daily routine), it is at the same time a metonymy (or, more specifically, a synecdoche). The woman went on to describe what the events meant to her, creating a new action metaphor—that of changing her life:

> I can't work in advertising anymore. I'm getting + doing something as a professional which is good for the world (and helps against hate, military and violence—in and by US and others).

It does not matter whether she really ended up doing what she wrote down. In the discursive context of her narrative this is a trope, a figure of speech that creates the vision of a new reality, a new life that aims to live up to the new after-9/11 state of the world. It combines the individual with the universal, connecting her life to the larger events that destroyed the pre-9/11 world. Its figurative power is derived from translating an abstract meaning into the concrete vision of someone who has come to believe she must change her life, her peculiar personal existence. In this sense, it is a unique linguistic expression, which "marks" a unique mental state, a state to whose existence the expression itself essentially contributes.

Other metaphors configure both a real scene and a mental state. This is the case in the story told by a man who, at the time of the attack, was working in his office in the World Finance Center across the street from the World Trade Center. He provides just one picture, cinematically speaking: one long and breathless take. While he is watching the burning tower from his window, the alarm is given to evacuate his building. And he starts, as he puts it, "running for my life," through smoke, shouts, police, and sirens. Even more detailed narrative imagery stands out in the story of a 73-year-old academic who tells how the attack has affected him:

> Work closed. A dozen or so unmarked cars (lights flashing on the dashboard) surrounded the glass building while I was fruitlessly trying to call on my cell phone and the land line. *This image is clear in my mind.* The cars were the F.B.I. They took over my workplace as headquarters, barricading the entrance, and posting 2 men w/LG [=with long guns] outside. They told us we could leave, but not come back. I walked back home, and work has been closed since.

Cinematically speaking, in this sequence the zoom of a metaphorical snapshot, as in the previous example, is extended along a chain of metonymies, a move reminiscent of further filmic techniques such as rapid cuts, cross-fades, close-ups, and rack focus (a shot during which the focus changes, shifting attention from one thing to another).

BEYOND STYLE

Aside from tropical and rhetorical devices and techniques such as metaphors, metonymies, and other imagery and its filmic montage, there are further linguistic resources to tackle and reconstruct traumatic experience. Linguistically, this is the level of style and textual or narrative composition. In fact, there is an extended literature on trauma narratives and the narrative-oriented study of trauma, in cultural and historical memory studies, literary theory, psychoanalysis, social sciences, postcolonial and gender/feminist studies. However—and this is my third observation regarding the 9/11 eyewitness accounts—there are also forms and features of style that seem more directed against any traditional idea of "style" and narrative composition, thus rejecting syntax and storyline altogether.

Recall the account of the woman walking near the towers when the first plane exploded, in which she speaks about her trouble organizing her everyday life and getting her nightmares under control. From here she goes on to write: "I am petrified, tired + not myself. I feel like I have been through a twilight zone episode. *Masks Military Police State Troopers Scary.*" Similar remarks are made by a 31-year-old woman answering the question what the attack means to the United States:

> What it means and what I wish it would mean are two different things, and what it means to the government is different from what it means to the population. It means: war peace attack isolation and [crossed out: or] an end to isolation justification being proven wrong a challenge a rallying cry a cry for help an excuse a means to an end

The continuous, chaotic, and overwhelming onslaught of impressions is often reported as one characteristic of traumatic experience. An essential part of posttraumatic stress disorder is the ongoing experience of shock, combined with the ongoing elusiveness of its components. Thus, postevent accounts of traumatic experience, which are structured by traditional principles of narrative coherence (such as, sequentiality, temporality, storyline), often create the feeling of inadequacy and distortion, rather than providing what is felt to be an authentic expression to one's traumatic experience, simply because the original experience of the traumatic event was all but coherent and well-ordered in the first place.

This is what the term "shock" essentially includes: the elusiveness of what constitutes it, the lack of structure and coherence. A staccato pacing of words without a recognizable pattern of narrative configuration as in the last sentence—or are we to read it as a staccato series of sentences?—seems to tell about exactly this dilemma. This, of course, is the dilemma of all trauma talk. But the break from traditional stylistic conventions manifested in this broken narrative seems to also suggest a way to go beyond it. Perhaps we can even understand it as a way to narrow the traumatic gap. It is as if it offers a form, as peculiar and stylistically unusual as it may be, that gives some sort of shape to the reality of an occurrence which by any normal standard ultimately remains inconceivable. Every expression, from war and peace to rallying cry and cry for help, offers a chain of metonymical and metaphorical extensions; each evokes splinters of experience, thought, and feeling; each potentially triggers a different stream of associations. And at the same time, the limitation and vagueness of any expression, if taken as a single and isolated statement, becomes evident. Like a kaleidoscope, it only needs a tiny shift and the picture changes entirely; this occurs without singling out one particular impression as center or periphery, as beginning or end, and, furthermore, without qualifying it as either perception or thought or emotion.

CAN THE TRAUMATIC GAP BE BRIDGED?

In his 1890 book, *The Principles of Psychology*, William James, in the chapter on "The stream of thoughts," wrote that "language works against our perception of truth" (p. 169). What he meant by this was that language tends always to give more stress to single terms (to substantives, in particular) than to both the relations and transitions among them and to the feelings that accompany our experience of them. While the stream of consciousness is essentially a process of continuous transition from one "substantive part" to the next, language (and we might add, especially the English language) revolves around nouns, continuously suggesting what James called "substantive conclusions." That is, language continuously fixates and, thus, isolates elements from this stream of perception and consciousness.

For James and many others, this interplay between language and the stream of thoughts and perceptions was problematic. It seemed to be responsible for the gap between language and some domains of our experience. These domains of experience and life do not lend themselves to "substantive conclusions" because they are too fleeting, malleable, and fragmentary. They are as vague and transient as is much of our existence. Human existence, as Heidegger put the matter in *Being and Time* (1962), is always "being-in-the-world," that is, it is being in the middle of a world of other things and relations. Thus human beings cannot be understood as fixed and isolated from their specific being in the world. However, for Heidegger, there is a tendency of language to do exactly this: fix and isolate. He saw this tendency predominantly within the language of science, whereas he considered the language of poetry as more open and sensitive to the particular, ephemeral, and entangled nature of the human condition.

Now, even if we are to accept this argument we should, however, not forget that it is the same ability of language to fixate and hold onto moments from an ongoing stream of consciousness that enables us to think at all. It enables us not only to step back and concentrate on experiences and thoughts, but also to reflect on emotions and moods. In this way, language allows us a number of things essential to our being in the world, namely: to interpret and give meaning to those experiences, thoughts, emotions, and moods; to communicate and engage in dialogue about their meanings; to reach out to others and open up to those who reach out to us. Without language, all of this would be impossible, or only possible in a very limited way. And without going beyond a representational notion of the relationship between language and experience it would be impossible, or only possible in a very limited way, to capture these phenomena.

But this is not to say that trauma accounts or trauma talk do not also represent something. So the question is, what do they represent? This is not an easy question to answer, and in order to sort it out we must be aware of some fundamental distinctions that are made by terms such as "traumatic event," "traumatic experience," "traumatic memory," and "trauma account." To begin, we must not confuse the representation of trauma with its effects, as in confusing a trauma account with the traumatic event itself. Moreover, the trauma account does not necessarily need to emerge from direct access to what originally was, or might have been, the traumatic event (an "event" that, by the way, is not always as accurately identifiable in time and space as it was for some on the morning of September 11). Nor does the trauma account emerge from any direct access to a traumatic experience of that event (note that the event itself is not identical with its experience; the same event can be experienced differently). Consider, furthermore, that we are talking about an experience in the past, something we usually call a memory. We therefore must keep in mind still another distinction: The representation given by a trauma account is that of a memory of a *past* experience, a memory that is articulated and, possibly, experienced again in the present. In other words, what is realized in the account is a process that does not affect the very traumatic event, nor its original experience, nor does it necessarily affect the memory of this experience; it only affects what Dominick LaCapra (2003) has called "the post-traumatic symptoms of that experience." Essentially, this is what the trauma account "represents," and in doing so, it also contributes at the same time to the discursive constitution of these symptoms. And while it is true that these posttraumatic symptoms may manifest themselves with or without language, "working them through" and possibly understanding them as present consequences of past events is hardly imaginable without the use of language. But, to add a final qualification, this is not to exclude the possibility that some posttraumatic symptoms "fade away" over time even without any trauma talk or "psychological debriefing," as mental health professionals have labeled it (e.g., Bisson, Jenkins, Alexander, & Bannister, 1997; Cannon, McKenzie, & Sims, 2003).

In a nutshell, then, any account of trauma as well as trauma talk is an event after the event. It is a memory report that is constrained and shaped as much by the present context in which it is told as it is by the past it claims to recall. Borrowing Mark Freeman's (2004) terms, we could say it oscillates between "the pressure of the past" and "the pressure of the present"—along with the language at hand.

Still, although the intricate dialectic interplay between experience and language, which we see unfolding in this relationship, enables us to make most of our experience the subject of conscious reflection and interpretation, it appears to fail in situations of extreme traumatic experience. As we know from many trauma survivors, the horror of such experience can be so total that it appears to exist beyond the reach of imagination, and it can only be distorted or falsified by attempts to bring it back to life. Articulated as a memory, and perhaps in the form of a story, the traumatic experience may indeed lose one of its essential qualities: the incomprehensibility of the original traumatic event. Extreme traumatic experiences, as already mentioned, are experiences of shock. They are chaotic, elusive, and paralyzing, and can sometimes lead to what Goldstein called uncontrolled "catastrophic reactions" in one's mind (Goldstein, 1995; Medved & Brockmeier, 2008). Perhaps phenomena like the dissolution of syntax and the absence of any punctuation (as in our last example: war peace attack isolation . . . a challenge a rallying cry a cry for help an excuse a means to an end), can be likened to Goldstein's catastrophic reaction. Perhaps it is us who witness here how the overwhelming experience of the crashing towers also "blew up" any conventional syntactic order.

It is not difficult to see how such experiences can escape, or even defy, language. To be more precise, it can escape and defy the experience-ordering potentials of a particular language: that of coherent narrative accounts, of stories in the classical Aristotelian sense. Aristotelian stories are narratives told according to the conventions of linearity, continuity, closure, and omniscience, conventions that have become canonical with 19th century realist writing. Since then they often have been taken as the quasi-natural condition of narrative. The cultural pressures to tell stories of this kind is kept up by educational, medical, legal, and other institutions and conventions, despite the fact that there are many different ways to make a story coherent. In fact, a variety of such forms are being used all the time, both in literary fiction and in everyday narrative discourse (Brockmeier, 2004).

Understandably, then, trauma victims often feel that such well-formed narrative templates are inadequate and too limited a format to be given to their experiences. As a consequence, some cannot or do not want to talk about their experiences. Typically, these experiences do not appear in trauma studies, nor did they appear in our 9/11 study. A few of these individuals may attempt to talk, only to become even more aware of the traumatic gap between their talking and what the talking is to be about: an experience that goes beyond all common and ordinary modes of experience, a break not just with a particular form of representation but with the very possibility of representation at all, a rupture not just with the way the world is depicted but a rupture within one's existence. It is, in fact, a rupture in one's being in the world.

Most of the accounts I have presented speak in one form or another to this experience of the limits, and by that I do not only mean the limits of language but also the limits of experience itself. Recent trauma research has emphasized that this rupture is essentially inherent to the traumatic experience itself, and that, at the core of this experience, is its failure to be represented in any common forms or modes of representation (Belau & Ramadanovic, 2002; Caruth, 1995, 1996; Hartman, 1994; LaCapra, 2001). In our culture such forms and modes of representation are typically defined in terms of Aristotelian concepts of narrative, be it oral, written, filmic, or performative. This is what I believe many trauma researchers have in mind when they refer to the essential incomprehensibility of the traumatic event. For example, when Cathy Caruth (1996, p. 154) speaks of "the force of its affront to understanding," she seems to be referring to these Aristotelian narrative forms and their obvious limits in capturing the elusive dimension of many traumatic experiences. As a result, increasing attention has been paid to trauma accounts (both in fiction and nonfiction) that reject realist conventions of narrative representation by using linguistic means associated with antirealist, experimental, and formally innovative types of narrative. Such non-Aristotelian forms of broken narrative do not claim to represent the original trauma; instead, they aim to embody its effects on perception, consciousness, and affect through their mode of narration. In a sense, they reevoke and reproduce the rupture within one's being in the world, bringing with it the force of its "affront to understanding"—without, however, pretending to ever reach the original event, let alone represent it.

How, then, can traumatic experiences be reembodied and reenacted? There are various linguistic resources that are pivotal here. For example, narrative techniques often mimic posttraumatic symptoms such "black outs" through interruptions, breaks, and voids in the narrative flow. Similarly, associated with such "wholes" there also are forms of narrative time construction that set up experiences of "fuzzy temporalities" (Herman, 2002). They are created through shock-like "anachronies" (the changing of a putative or expected temporal order of events), the stretching or flexing of time (to make it faster or slower), ellipses and repetitions. "When a reader," as Kacandes (2005, p. 618) argues, "makes the connection between such textual features and trauma she is engaged in literary-historical witnessing to the trauma of the text." Furthermore, in the quoted 9/11 eyewitness accounts we find stylistic-tropical and scriptural-graphic resources to recreate effects of shock. Sometimes people reenact personal catastrophes, nightmares, anxiety, depression, and dissociation in very imagistic language, and talk can take on a strong expressive and performative form (Langellier, 2001). In 20th-century modernist literature, a broad spectrum of all these linguistic forms has developed, leaving its impact on holocaust testimonies, memoirs, novels, and poems by Paul Celan, Charlotte Delbo, Imre Kertész, Ruth Klüger, Jorge Semprun, Martin Amis, W.G. Sebald, and others. Comparable marks have been left on the visual arts (Rapaport, 2002), music (especially in the Schönberg tradition; Schultz, 2006); and cinematography (e.g., as in films by Ingmar Bergman).

THE CONVENTIONAL PLOT:
DETRAUMATIZING THE TRAUMATIC GAP

It is true that irrespective of such narrative resources, the events of September 11 have been reported, recounted, and endlessly retold in quite traditional ways. Given their many layers of political, ideological, and military meanings, this is hardly surprising. Remember the cultural canonicity of Hollywood disaster films. Earlier I mentioned some of the interests shaping these stories, and how they affected my own reluctance and ambivalence not only with respect to the eyewitness accounts but, in fact, to the entire research project. While in those days I found myself at a loss for making sense of the many bewildering and heartbreaking aspects of the September events, I was also confronted with a robust and seemingly ubiquitous master narrative in the aftermath of those events which claimed to provide a most coherent explanation. A similar case in point comes from the documentary film "9/11" by the Naudet brothers (which aired on CBS on March 10, 2002, as well as on TV stations around the world on the first anniversary of the attacks). In his analysis of this highly acclaimed documentary, literary critic and trauma theorist Stef Craps (2007) explains how the film seeks to reorganize its disturbing footage (which was shot primarily within one of the burning World Trade Towers while the other is collapsing) according to a most conventional narrative plot model. This attempt to conventionally reorganize, Craps argues, results in a fundamental tension between the cameraman's testimony, that reveals "an abysmal crisis" of order and meaning occurring at the scene, and "the desire to bring this crisis under control." This control is exerted by imposing a story line on the events following a young probationary New York firefighter, a "probie," as he grows through the catastrophe into a true man and American hero.

> The filmmakers attempt to mitigate the traumatic potential of their unique atrocity footage by sanitizing it and integrating it into a Hollywood-style coming-of-age drama, tracing a probationary fire-fighter's perilous journey from innocence to experience. Thus, the focus shifts

from a disorienting and overwhelming sense of loss to comforting, ideologically charged notions of heroism and community that perpetuate an idealized national self-image and come to function as a moral justification for retaliation. (Craps, 2007, p. 185)

Craps shows that the film's "drive to obtain mastery over trauma by rendering it legible in terms of existing cultural codes" does not entirely succeed. In a few scenes, the footage of chaos, panic, angst, and dying, although heavily censored and "sanitized," becomes so overwhelming that it defies the imposed "heroic" storyline.

[The] harrowing images drive home the traumatic impact of events in excess of our conceptual categories and frames of reference. Besides filming the horrific events themselves from up close, the camera also captures the look of bewilderment, disbelief, incomprehension, fear and powerlessness on the faces of people caught in the most appalling disaster. The retrospective interviews with the film-makers and the fire-fighters which are interspersed with this footage confirm these responses. Gedeon and Jules [Naudet] recall the inability of the passersby and the fire-fighters to believe what was happening before their eyes: "[w]alking to the World Trade Center, passing by these people, filming their astonishment. Eyes saying: this is not happening?" (Gedeon); "I was seeing the look on the fire-fighters [sic]. It was not fear, it was: what's going on? Disbelief. That made me panic a little bit. That made me panic" (Jules). Several fire-fighters stress the complete unexpectedness of what took place ("we'd never experienced something like this before") and the impossibility of bringing the situation under control ("what do we do, what do we do for this?"). These reactions are clearly symptomatic of trauma, understood as a sudden, unexpected, and overwhelming experience that escapes one's grasp—whether conceptual or physical—and, as a result, keeps haunting one. (Craps, 2007, pp. 186–87)

Craps's analysis demonstrates that the film, for all its investment in a classical realist narrative aesthetic and its attempts to "detraumatize" September 11, still remains haunted by traumatic experiences that exceed and break down accustomed habits of narration and visualization, including those ones it tries to impose upon these experiences itself.

SUBJECTIVITY AND THE LANGUAGE OF SCIENCE

Is it possible, then, that a similar sense of inadequacy and contradiction between experience and its representation was triggered in those who completed the 9/11 survey questionnaire by the questionnaire itself? I already pointed out that the study was first and foremost interested in people's memory capacity, and not in their personal or subjective reactions or, put differently, in their meaning making under extreme circumstances. The questionnaire was couched in a highly technical, even bureaucratic language, as is typical of survey studies of this kind. And what's more, in this way the survey imposed the same style on the answers of participants, many of whom still under shock and mourning the loss of friends and colleagues.

What the style and composition of the questionnaire embodied was an interest in decontextualized and fragmented information, with a focus on exact numeric details: "What airline or airlines had planes hijacked? How many from each airline?" and "For each airline, what was their intended route, departure, arrival?" The entire questionnaire represented a type of knowledge and memory that was deemed to be particularly appropriate for statistical elaboration (an elaboration that was to also include the "data" provided by the questionnaires of the follow-up studies). In a sense, the questionnaire constructed exactly the type of knowledge and memory that it was after. What it did not show was any interest in how the eyewitnesses tried to come to terms with their experiences. Since the language of the questionnaire and the accompanying material wasn't meant to capture traumatic experiences or emotion, it would have been incapable of doing so. And so we encounter another gap between language and experience: the gap between the language of what is understood as science and the subjectivity of human beings who are attempting to come to terms with existentially disturbing experiences. Once again, these phenomena are left outside the edifice of scientific psychology; they are in all their "ambiguity and unwieldiness . . . relegated to philosophers and poets, those more willing to enter these dense thickets of the human experience" (Freeman, 2005).

After reading these accounts, admittedly with my own ambivalence, I couldn't help but wonder if some of the commentaries given by the participants, after they had gone through dozens of its information-centered questions, also reflected something else. Perhaps there existed an unease, or maybe an emerging suspicion, in those who might have sensed that the study was not interested in their true experiences at all. In other words, were we to understand the radical tone of many accounts as a protest, even if unintended or unconscious, against a research design that was capable of asking dozens of questions without touching on the existential significance of this experience for those who had it "happen in their faces"? Could it be, then, that some of the short narratives, squeezed into the questionnaire (remember that a significant number of the accounts went well beyond the instruction of "one brief paragraph") were also to be read as a protest against a kind of research that only seemed to be interested in the witnesses' traumatic experience? That was only interested in those experiences in as far as they fell into categories of cognitive operations of which the designers of the study believed human memory to consist? Could it be that some of the participants might have felt like memory information donors—much as pupils felt in "Hailsham," the obscure educational establishment in Kazuo Ishiguro's novel *Never Let Me Go,* where children are brought up to believe they are special, while their entire education comes down to the sole purpose of using them as organ donors?

I began this essay by stating that there are many ways to tackle the relationship between language and experience; one is to listen to people who have had certain experiences that they feel escape their words and, at times, escape all words. Apparently, in the case of the 9/11 memory study it was not so much the failure of words in general, but of particular words—the language of "cognitive science"—that failed to reach the experience of those whose memory it claimed to investigate. However, as we saw, this is not the entire story. There were more words, words provided by the eyewitnesses, that were different. These were words that belonged to the language of traumatic experience, articulated in what I have called a "narrative surplus": allowing us to better understand what the traumatic gap is about, how people are aware of it, and how they attempt to bridge it, coping with experiences that have shattered more than just conventions of narrative and, for that matter, the language of "science."

Examining this narrative surplus, I have offered three observations. On the one hand, they emphasize different aspects of the inadequacy of the language used to describe the events and their meaning in personal and emotional terms. On the other hand, these observations emphasize some attempts (and their linguistic resources) to narrow or, at least, express the sense of this inadequacy. These attempts include forms and features of style and narrative composition that seem more directed against any traditional idea of style, syntax, and storyline. All of this, I have argued, might reflect not so much the fundamental limits or flaws of language in "expressing" or "representing" traumatic experience, but the very essence of this experience and its memory. Human experience and language are in many different ways intimately mingled and, at times, even fused. But none of these many different ways can be understood by means of a representational notion of language. Such a notion would assume that language merely represents (or depicts, mirrors, expresses, or reflects) a non- or pre-semiotically immediate reality. In contrast, the nonrepresentational Wittgensteinian understanding underlying my point of view conceives of language and other human sign systems as always already part of the cultural fabric that we consider to be our reality. Language, in this view, is not only inherent to our reality, but constitutive of our being in the world.

I see a similar nonrepresentational view emerging in recent trauma theory. By understanding trauma as a fundamentally overwhelming, incomprehensible, and elusive experience, a number of researchers and scholars have come to reject the idea that the traumatic experience can be and should be transformed into a coherent story. It is in line with these considerations that I have proposed traumatic experience as a break not just with a particular form of representation but with the very possibility of representation at all. This representational break culminates in the breakdown of narrativity. The traumatic gap between language and experience does not just reflect a rupture with the way the world is depicted but with the existential basis of human meaning making. What it reveals is a rupture in one's being in the world.

NOTES

1. Although I have a number of reservations regarding the conceptual and methodological set-up of psychological research projects of this kind—I will say more about it in what follows—I am of course grateful for the generous invitation to study the material of the project, having unlimited access to its rich data collections, and the possibility to use frameworks of interpretation that are different from, or alternative to, those underlying the design of the project.
2. This tradition was initiated in 1977 by cognitive psychologists Roger Brown and James Kulik who studied the impact of large-scale traumatic events on individual memory. Brown and Kulik used the assassination of President Kennedy as the source of their research, which focused on the quality and accuracy of memories of witnesses. The assumption underlying this tradition was that sudden and emotionally salient events imprint themselves in memory to a degree that they create a unique mnemotic experience like that of the images on a flashbulb photograph. Summarizing their research philosophy, the "National 9/11 Memory Consortium" stated (on its website) that "[t]he terrorist attack of 9/11 is not only a significantly traumatic event that qualifies for this type of research, but may be considered, by the nature of the scale, intensity, and breadth of its effect, to be the definitive case study of memory for a public, traumatic event." Accordingly, after the initial survey of September 2001, two follow-up surveys were conducted, the first at 1 year and the second at 3 years after the attacks.

REFERENCES

Belau, L., & Ramadanovic, P. (Eds.). (2002). *Topologies of trauma: Essays on the limit of knowledge and memory*. New York: Other Press.

Bisson, J. I., Jenkins, P. L., Alexander, J., & Bannister, C. (1997). Randomized controlled trial of psychological debriefing for victims of acute burn trauma. *British Journal of Psychiatry, 171*, 78–81.

Brockmeier, J. (2002). Ineffable experience. *The Journal for Consciousness Studies, 9*, 79–95.

Brockmeier, J. (2004). What makes a story coherent? In A. U. Branco & J. Valsiner (Eds.), *Communication and metacommunication in human development* (pp. 285–306). Greenwich, CT: Information Age Publishing.

Brockmeier, J. (in press). Reaching for meaning: Human agency and the narrative imagination. *Theory and Psychology*.

Brown, R., & Kulik, J. (1977). Flashbulb memories. *Cognition, 5*, 73–99.

Cannon, M., McKenzie, K., & Sims, A. (2003). Psychological debriefing is a waste of time. *British Journal of Psychiatry, 183*, 12–14.

Caruth, C. (Ed.). (1995). *Trauma: Explorations in memory.* Baltimore: Johns Hopkins University Press.

Caruth, C. (1996). *Unclaimed experience: Trauma, narrative, and history.* Baltimore: Johns Hopkins University Press.

Craps, S. (2007). Conjuring trauma: The Naudet brothers' 9/11 documentary. *Canadian Review of American Studies, 37,* 185–204.

Derrida, J. (2005). *Sovereignties in question: The poetics of Paul Celan* (T. Dutoit & O. Pasane, Eds.). New York: Fordham University Press.

Freeman, M. (2004). Charting the narrative unconscious: Cultural memory and the challenge of autobiography—Response to commentaries. In M. Bamberg & M. Andrews (Eds.), *Considering counter-narratives: Narrating, resisting, making sense* (pp. 341–350). Amsterdam & Philadelphia: John Benjamins.

Freeman, M. (2005, April). Science and story. Talk at the conference *Methods in Dialog,* Hemingford, Cambridge, UK (Centre for Narrative Research and the London East Research Institute, University of East London).

Goldstein, K. (1995). *The organism: A holistic approach to biology derived from pathological data in man.* New York: Zone Books. (Original work published 1934)

Hartman, G. H. (Ed.). (1994). *Holocaust remembrance: The shape of memory.* Oxford, UK: Blackwell.

Heidegger, M. (1962). *Being and time.* New York: Harper & Row.

Herman, D. (2002). *Story logic: Problems and possibilities of narrative.* Lincoln, NE: University of Nebraska Press.

James, W. (1981). *The principles of psychology (Vol 1).* Cambridge, MA: Harvard University Press. (Original work published 1890)

Kacandes, I. (2005). Trauma theory. In D. Herman, M. Jahn, & M.-L. Ryan (Eds.), *The Routledge encyclopedia of narrative theory* (pp. 615–619). London: Routledge.

LaCapra, D. (2001). *Writing history, writing trauma.* Baltimore: Johns Hopkins University Press.

LaCapra, D. (2003, May). *The consequences of witnessing trauma.* Paper presented at the Colloquium Narrative Medicine, Columbia University, New York City, College of Physicians and Surgeons.

Langellier, K. (2001). "You're marked": Breast cancer, tattoo and the narrative performance of identity. In J. Brockmeier & D. Carbaugh (Eds.), *Narrative and identity: Studies in autobiography, self, and culture* (pp. 145–184). Amsterdam and Philadelphia: John Benjamins.

Medved, M. I., & Brockmeier, J. (2004). Making sense of traumatic experiences: Telling your life with Fragile X syndrome. *Qualitative Health Research, 14,* 741–759.

Medved, M. I., & Brockmeier, J. (2008). Talking about the unthinkable: Brain injuries and the "catastrophic reaction." In L.-C. Hydén & J. Brockmeier (Eds.), *Health, illness and culture: Broken narratives* (pp. 54–72). New York: Routledge.

Rapaport, H. (2002). Representation, history, and trauma: Abstract art after 1945. In L. Belau & P. Ramadanovic (Eds.), *Topologies of trauma: Essays on the limit of knowledge and memory* (pp. 233–250). New York: Other Press.

Schultz, W.-A. (2006). Avantgarde und Trauma. Die Musik des 20. Jahrhunderts und die Erfahrung der Weltkriege [Avant-garde and trauma. The music of 20th century and the experience of the world wars]. *Lettre International, 71,* 92–97.

Sontag, S. (2003). *Regarding the pain of others.* London: Hamish Hamilton.

Thomson, D. (2006, April 30). Films of infamy. *The New York Times,* p. 15.

3 Broken and Vicarious Voices in Narratives

Lars-Christer Hydén

INTRODUCTION

By working on that one story of mine every day—even small amounts at a time—I hoped I'd be able to tell people about this illness and overcome it. I've already worked on the story of my illness for three years. Writing about and studying myself is my way of thinking, keeping busy, working at something. It reassures me, so I keep at it. By doing it again and again (I don't know how many times I've rewritten this over the years), my speaking ability has improved. I really do speak better now and can remember words that were scattered into bits and pieces by my head wound. By training myself (through thinking and writing) I've gotten to the point where I can carry on a conversation—at least about simple, everyday matters. (Luria, 1973, p. 85)

Zasetsky, a Soviet soldier, was hit in the head by a German bullet in 1944. The bullet destroyed portions of his brain, and as a consequence he lost the ability to create order in his life. His past became impenetrable and his daily life was split into parts that lacked any internal coherence. By devoting effort for decades to writing and speaking, Zasetsky could finally begin to find his own voice again. He could slowly patch together his shattered world into an integral whole, and thus begin to regain his life and to create order in it.

For Zasetsky this was only possible with the help he received from his doctor, who aided him in putting things into context and creating an entirety—a task that was impossible for Zasetsky to do by himself. Dr. Luria could function as a vicarious supporting voice, by lending form to what Zasetsky could not connect on his own. We will come back to Zasetsky, Aleksandr Luria, and their relationship again later in this chapter.

Zasetsky and his fate illustrate the issue and the set of problems that are the focus of this chapter. What happens when a person is unable, due to illness or injury, to formulate his or her own voice and communicate his or her own experiences—and becomes dependent on having the help of another person who functions as a sort of vicarious voice? The vicarious voice can be that of another family member, or a doctor, or some other care person. The central question is how the relationship between the person who has lost his or her voice and the vicarious voice looks. Is it possible to maintain a lost voice against the vicarious voice? Can the vicarious voice subordinate a weak voice? What happens in an extreme case where a person completely lacks a voice, and perhaps never actually had one?

I will discuss this kind of question first against a background of autobiographical narration. Then I will introduce the concepts of sounding and authorial voices and the relationship between these voices. Of special interest to me are cases when a person is unable, due to illness or disease, to give voice to his or her specific experiences and point of view, and someone else acts as a vicarious voice. I am going to illustrate this set of problems by choosing three cases that represent different relationships between the voices and different ways of creating a vicarious voice.

AUTOBIOGRAPHICAL NARRATION

A common and strong argument among many philosophers and psychologists is that it is through creating, elaborating, revising, and scrutinizing narratives of our own lives that we come to develop and possess an identity and a sense of ourselves as persons—a sense of self. Jens Brockmeier and Donal Carbaugh argue that "narrative proves to be a supremely appropriate means for the exploration of the self or, more precisely, the construction of selves in cultural contexts of time and space" (2001, p. 15). In other words, it is by telling and listening to stories that we get a chance not only to understand ourselves and other persons, but it is also through this process that we *can* construct a self.

Among philosophers, the American feminist Marya Schechtman argues in the same vein that a person "creates his identity by forming an autobiographical narrative—a story of his life" (Schechtman, 1996, p. 93). According to her it is also important to be in possession of a full and "explicit narrative to develop fully as a person" (p. 119). Many philosophers and social scientists have argued for similar positions.

For most of these researchers, the type of narrative of interest is autobiographical stories. Jerome Bruner writes that autobiographical stories are produced when a "narrator, in the here and now, takes upon himself or herself the task of describing the progress of the protagonist in the there and then, one who happens to share his name" (2001, p. 27). In other words, we tell autobiographical stories about ourselves and our experiences—stories that are supposed to be true, at least in the sense that we actually experienced both the events and the persons that figure in the stories.

In this perspective, autobiographical narratives are connected to a unique individual—the person who not only tells about the experiences but also is supposed to have had them and consequently own these experiences. If we are telling stories instead about experiences that someone else is supposed to have had, we are telling a story about vicarious experiences (for the term, see Labov, 1972).

In other words, the notion of autobiographical narration rests on a strong connection between the individual and his or her experiences, stories, and identity. This notion is further not only rooted in our cultural conception of what an individual is, but also of what he or she ought to be. Many authors interested in the historical emergence of the autobiographical narrative mode often argue for a strong historical connection between the emerging literary autobiography and the emergence of Western individualism and even egalitarian individualism (Weintraub 1978; Gusdorf, 1980; Eakin, 2001).

What happens in situations where the teller or author has some form of communicative disability leading to an inability to fulfill the roles of teller *of* the story, and narrator and character *in* the story? In short, what happens when we are unable tell stories? Or, when we as tellers are unable to create, elaborate, revise, and scrutinize our own lives by telling stories? Does such a person lack an identity and a sense of self?

SEVERAL VOICES: SOUNDING, AUTHORIAL, AND VICARIOUS

One way to discuss this question is to start from the idea that autobiographical narration, just like all other forms of narration, is based on having events related from a special perspective. In the case of autobiographical narration this is accomplished by the fact that the narrating individual relates his or her own experiences and events and is himself or herself the main person in the narration. One way of talking about both the delivery of the narrative and its perspective is to use the concept of *voice,* which is associated with Michail Bakhtin (Bakhtin, 1984), a Russian specialist in comparative literature.

Voice can, in this connection, refer to two different but related phenomena. The first one is *the sounding voice,* that is, the voice that others can hear in the sounds it produces. Every sounding voice is personal, since its acoustic image is unique.

The second one is the *authorial voice,* the "authorship" of the special experiences and special perspective of the world and of life that are connected to the individual and his or her biography. It is authorial because here it is not the acoustic image that is in focus, but rather the process by which the thought is clad in words—to use a metaphor of the Russian psychologist Lev Vygotsky (1987)—and thereby can sound.

The authorial voice brings out, links together, and communicates that which is the individual's special experience and perspective of the world. The authorial voice starts out as an intention and a gesture, and must be clad in words in order to be communicated. Memories, thoughts, and associations can all exist in compressed form, but in order for them to be communicated they must be converted into (for example) the form of language (Brockmeier, 2008). Otherwise they remain inaccessible both to the individual and to others. In this sense the authorial voice is not given, but rather constitutes a process by which it is formulated through the words and their organization.

Both the sounding and the authorial voices can be silenced. We can lose the physical capacity to use our voices—but despite that retain the authorial voice and communicate with the aid of, for example, written words. It is also possible that another person loans his or her physical voice to function as a vicarious voice. The vicarious voice may thus utter words that are unfamiliar to the vicarious voice, because they constitute another person's authorial voice. Finally, a synthetic or artificial voice can function as a vicarious sounding voice.

The sounding voice can also be silenced for political reasons, because one is not permitted to make oneself heard. This may not be because of the voice itself—although examples of this exist too—but rather because of the perspective and the experiences that the sounding voice can convey. The silence of the sounding voice forces the personal perspective to go undercover and live in hiding. But even the silenced voice can find a vicarious voice that can convey perceptions of that which is forbidden when someone else with greater freedom tells about the experiences.

The authorial voice can be weak, in development, or—in the extreme—go silent or fall apart. The authorial voice is created from the dialogue with other people, and then grows forth as part of an inner dialogue. This means that the child develops its authorial voice together with its parents, to then become the bearer of his or her own voice. The adult helps the child to narrate by acting as an example, by showing how a narrative should be constructed—which events and perceptions should be emphasized, and how to formulate a point.

This issue has been discussed extensively by authors like Elinor Ochs and Lisa Capps in their book *Living Narrative* (2001), by Peggy Miller (1994), Robyn Fivush (1994), and several other researchers. A similar situation is faced when, for instance, younger family members communicate with older family members afflicted by Alzheimer's disease. The younger family members have to support the conversation in order to guide it forward (Sabat, 2001).

This is also a kind of relationship that is found in institutional contexts characterized by strong asymmetric relationships between the parties. It can be a matter of something like a strong asymmetry in knowledge of law, when a lawyer represents a client either by telling the court the client's story or by leading the client with his questions to communicate the "right" story for the members of the jury.

The same type of knowledge asymmetry is present in the meeting between a doctor and patient, in which the doctor organizes and sums up the patient's reports and narrations into a medical narration that then becomes the basis for the continued clinical treatment (Cicourel, 1975; Mishler, 1984). When patients lose their abilities to formulate their own authorial voices, for example as a result of Alzheimer's disease or some neurological trauma, the doctor and other care staff must function as their vicarious voices. Similar situations appear in psychotherapeutic relationships when the client has somehow lost the ability to formulate his or her own authorial voice (see, e.g., Hydén, 1995; Josselson, 2004).

The silencing or breakdown of the authorial voice is something that often occurs in diseases or injuries of the central nervous system resulting in difficulties using language and in other cognitive faculties, for example memory. The authorial voice can also break down because the person who was to formulate it is not psychologically capable of maintaining memories, perceptions, and experiences. The individual voice is broken, and lacks an inner focus.

When the authorial voice is broken, experiences and memories cannot be turned into words that the physical voice can speak. Often the sounding voice remains, but it lacks words and direction. When the authorial voice cannot find the words, it cannot find order and coherence. Both voices fall silent, or utter words that lack a communicative intention.

What is needed in this situation is therefore not just a vicarious voice, since the problem is not primarily one of communicating sound. The problem is that the authorial voice does not function, and thus needs a *vicarious authorial voice*, in other words someone who can help formulate the thoughts, memories, experiences, and intentions that the injured person cannot formulate for himself or herself. It is a process of voicing, albeit not only physically but also psychologically.

THE VICARIOUS AUTHORIAL VOICE

Functioning as a vicarious voice involves entering into a relationship with another person, both with the physical person and his or her physical voice, and with his or her authorial voice—with the person's way of perceiving the world.

When a person loans his or her physical voice to another person who is not capable of using his or her voice, it is a situation in which there already exists a prepared text that the vicarious voice conveys. An analogous situation would be that of an actor who is to transform a drama from a text to a play.

Acting as a "sounding box"—to use Erving Goffman's concept (1981)— always involves having the vicarious voice establish a relationship with the text that is to be conveyed physically. A text must be interpreted, for example, by emphasizing certain words, using others quickly or slowly, with or without a dialect, and so on. In other words, the sounding voice can only function as a living voice, as seen from an analysis of the text in question. A text can only be analyzed in a meeting of the vicarious voice's own authorial voice with the text's authorial voice, and from that meeting the vicarious sounding voice can find its tone. The alternative to this is a synthetic voice that is as indifferent to the words as it is monotonous.

When a person lacks the ability to form his or her own authorial voice, it is not only the sounds that are missing, but perhaps more importantly the words that "clothe" the authorial voice—words which are organized, for instance, into a narrative. The thought, the perception, the memories lack not only the sounding aspect, but also the words that transform the thought or the memory into something communicable. This means that a vicarious voice not only has to loan out the sounding voice, but also act as an organizing voice. The vicarious voice thus attains a double function, both as "sounding box" and as "author" (Goffman, 1981).

When we retell what another person has said or done, we can do it in one of two ways. Either we imitate the person and thus repeat the words literally, or else we can render indirectly what the other person said, by telling it in our own words. This presupposes an analysis of the other person's speech and actions, in order to clothe them in our own words.

Similarly, someone who is to function as a vicarious authorial voice must remain analytical. In order to formulate another person's voice it is necessary to try to understand what that person wants to say or is trying to say—to try to identify the original gesture and intention. In other words, the vicarious person must use his or her own analytical abilities to understand the first person's communicative gesture.

Thus a symmetrical relationship is established between the voices. The injured person's voice—both the sounding and the authorial voices—are weak and have difficulty asserting themselves on their own. The vicarious voice, however, is not only intact, but it also reconstructs the other person's authorial voice. Even though we can imagine a dialogue between the weak voice and the vicarious voice, there is always the possibility that the vicarious voice will incorporate the other person's voice into his or her own voice.

I will discuss below how the relationship between these voices—the actual ones and the potential ones—can be configured.

THREE CASES

In the following I want to discuss three different kinds of relationships between an authorial voice and a vicarious authorial voice.

The first case is when a person may be able to talk and produce narrative, but for various reasons the narrative is fragmentary and threatens to become unintelligible to listeners. For that reason the narrative may need supplementing, support, and comments, for instance in a second person perspective. Dorothy, a victim of a hit and run accident that left her with severe brain trauma, illustrates this. The focus is on a situation in which she tells her story jointly with her nurse. In a second case we have a person who is unable to produce a narrative without support, due to a condition like severe aphasic problems (problems with using language). In this case the vicarious voice has the possibility of supporting the first person narration by adding a third-person perspective. We will meet Zasetsky again, the Soviet soldier who got a German bullet in his brain in 1943, and who worked with his neurologist Aleksandr Luria for more than 25 years trying to understand his new brain.

The third case is an extreme one where a person is totally unable to use language at all; this includes cases where the person has never been able to use language or may be unconscious. In this case the vicarious voice has to substitute not only the function of actual physical production of an autobiographical narrative, but also substitute for narrator and character, including the invention of a sort of first person perspective. I will exemplify this discussion from philosopher Hilde Nelson's portrayal of her sister Clara, who was never able to tell an autobiographical narrative, but who had a caring family that spun stories around her, constructing her identity.

In these cases the vicarious voice has three different relationships to the person with communicative dysfunctions. The vicarious voice *supports*, *supplements*, or *substitutes* the voice of the affected person.

Supportive narration

Brain trauma or disease may affect the ability to use language, and as a consequence the ability to tell stories. Various problems can emerge, depending on the type of pathology. To what extent cognitive functions are involved is of special importance, like for instance in memory or if the injuries affect the linguistic ability in a narrower sense.

It is of course possible to think about these problems in various ways. The literary theorist Kay Young and the neurologist Jeffrey Saver have identified what they call four different types of dysnarration due to neurological problems (Young & Saver, 2001). Their idea is to identify specific narrative problems and relate these to neurological pathologies. The first type of dysnarration is what they call arrested narration.

Arrested narration is an inability to create new narrative due to a general amnesia; among other things this means that the person is unable to form new memories after the trauma and to tell stories about recent events. Persons with lesions on their frontal lobe structures also exhibit uncontrolled narration. That is, they have no ability to self-monitor and as a result tell stories unconstrained by memories of actual events. This type of narrative is often thought of as confabulatory (although for a somewhat different interpretation of confabulation, see Örulv & Hydén, 2006). Young and Save write about these persons that they "offer an unrivalled glimpse at the power of the human impulse to narrate."

Individuals with damage to their bilateral ventromedial frontal lobe have access to their autobiographical memories but have problems with inhibiting their immediate responses, for instance to requests. As a consequence they fail to construct and explore narrative space. This means that they cognitively fail to set up several possible answers with different consequences. As a consequence they don't make a choice between several possible narratives, but choose their first response. As a result these persons *undernarrate*.

Finally, individuals with lesions to their dorsolateral frontal cortices have problems constructing and organizing meaning in ongoing activities. This means that they are basically unable to construct narratives about their experiences—a sort of *denarration*.

This taxonomy of dysnarrations lets us observe the fact that there are connections between brain functions, traumas, and pathologies, and the way we are able to tell stories—in the same way that neurologists from Kurt Goldstein and Aleksandr Luria to Oliver Sacks have suggested (see Goldstein, 1948; Sacks, 1985; Medved & Brockmeier, 2008). At the same time, this taxonomy rests on a decontextualization of the story-telling individuals. We do not know anything, especially, about the interaction between the examining doctor and the patient. Of particular interest are of course the way the examining doctor makes a request for a story, what his or her expectations are concerning the form of the narrative, and whether and in what way they support storytelling. Steven Sabat has pointed out that people afflicted by Alzheimer's disease need constant support by others in order to be able to keep track of their conversational topics, as well as help finding words (Sabat, 2001). If the other is nonsupportive, the affected person may appear less capable than he or she actually is. The same holds true for people with other types of neurological diseases or traumas.

Thus it is interesting to focus on the interaction between narrators and listeners, especially if the narrator is a patient and the listener is a medical doctor or some other type of professional. The following example comes from material collected at an activity center mainly for persons with brain traumas. (Eleonor Antelius, doctoral student at Linköping University has collected this material. She has kindly let me use this example from her vast video recorded material. All names have been changed.) The majority of the visitors to the center are between 20 and 60 years of age, and many of them have been in severe car accidents. One of these persons is Margret. She is around 45 years and has been in contact with the activity center for about 5 years. One of the nurses working with Margret is named Dorothy and she has known Margret for about 4 years. For an extended period, Eleonor did her fieldwork at the center, videofilming everyday life (Antelius, 2007). One afternoon Dorothy asks Margret if she has told Eleonor why she is in a wheelchair.

> Dorothy: have you told Eleonor, who is sitting over there ((points towards Eleonor)) why you are in a wheelchair?
> Margret: no
> Eleonor: no
>   I don't think so
> Margret: car accidents
> Eleonor: accidents?
>   more than one?
> Margret: ((nods)) two
> Eleonor: two?
>   ((Margret looks at Dorothy))
> Dorothy: you had almost recovered from the first one
>   Trained yourself
>   When did it happen?
> Margret: one year
> Dorothy: one year between the accidents?
> Margret: then the second one happened
> Dorothy: were you in a car both times?
> Margret: yeah
> Dorothy: yes, I thought you rode a motorcycle
> Margret: car
> Dorothy: yes it was a car.
>   But you didn't drive yourself?
> Margret: yes: the second time
> Dorothy: you drove the second time?
> Margret: on my way to ((xxx))
> Dorothy: on your way to?
> Margret: my work
> Dorothy: your job yes
> Margret: ((xxx)) who drove were drunk
> Dorothy: he was drunk yes
> Margret: ((xxx))
> Dorothy: did you start your job at night?
>   ((Margret nods))
>   yes you did work the night shift
> Margret: always

Dorothy suggests that Margret should tell the story about her car accidents. Margret starts doing this using a very reduced vocabulary. She for instance starts by saying "car accidents"; the plural form of "accidents" indicates that she has suffered more than one accident. In response to a question by Eleonor, Margret can specify that she suffered two accidents, but then she apparently cannot elaborate the answer and turns to Dorothy, who interprets this as a request for help. Dorothy helps Margret by putting the events in order; she had almost recovered from the first accident when another car hit her.

Between Dorothy and Margret a sort of joint narration quickly evolves. Either Dorothy puts supportive questions to Margret, who can then fill in more specific information about an event, or Margret uses a short word or phrase (something which is more apparent in Swedish), and Dorothy elaborates on this by posing expanding questions. A closer look at the conversation shows that Dorothy is generally familiar with Margret's story. She knows at least the general outline of the events that put Margret into her wheelchair. She also knows the important points in Dorothy's story, for instance that her second accident occurred just when she had recovered from her first accident. She was on her way to her night shift job, was hit by a drunken driver, and bore no responsibility for the accident.

In her supportive utterances Dorothy address Margret in the second person, for instance, "I thought *you* rode a motorcycle" and "*You* drove the second time?" These utterances are incorporated into the unfolding narrative and partly substitute for the first person perspective that Dorothy has problems articulating on her own.

Dorothy's use of the second-person address form at the same time makes it clear that she subordinates her narrative contributions to Margret's story. Dorothy apparently does not want to add any personal story elements outside of what Margret herself wants to tell.

Dorothy's vicarious voice enters into a dialogue with Margret's own voice. Dorothy takes hints from Margret in order to be able to help her to reconstruct her experiences. Dorothy keeps the narrative close to Margret's own memories, her perspective on the events, and her evaluation of them. In that sense, Dorothy's vicarious voice basically supports Margret's own authorial voice.

Supplementary Narration

> I'm in a kind of fog all the time, like a heavy half-sleep. My memory's a blank. I can't think of a single word. All that flashes through my mind are some images, hazy visions that suddenly appear and just as suddenly disappear, giving way to fresh images,. But I simply can't understand or remember what these mean. Whatever I do remember is scattered, broken down into disconnected bits and pieces. That's why I react so abnormally to every word and idea, every attempt to understand the meaning of words. (Luria, 1973, pp. 11–12)

The person writing this, as mentioned earlier, is a former soldier called Zasetsky. He is also known as Z; as readers we never get to know his first name or if this really is his name. To Zasetsky the world is shattered. It fell to pieces at the same moment as his brain fell to pieces. He cannot connect all the events and impressions that constitute the world because he is unable to tell a story; his linguistic abilities are limited as a result of his brain trauma. His world had turned into a broken narrative.

Zasetsky was hit by a German bullet in the left side of the brain—in the parieto-occipital area—on March 2, 1943. He received emergency treatment and was then brought to a rehabilitation hospital in the Ural. At this hospital, he met Aleksandr Luria, a neurologist, in May 1943. Due to his brain injury Zasetsky lost most of his ability to use language and became unable to create continuity in his experiences, to perceive meaning in what he saw and experienced.

As a result of extensive and intensive rehabilitation Zasetsky slowly began to be able understand words, combinations of words, and also to write. Aleksandr Luria and other persons encouraged Zasetsky to write and in fact to keep a diary. During the following 25 years, Zasetsky wrote over 3,000 diary pages. Over and over he tried to write about his injury, his painstaking rehabilitation, and how he experienced the world.

The texts that Zasetsky produced turned out to be fragments centered on events in his life and his present situation. Many years later Aleksandr Luria edited some of the diary material, added his own comments, and published these as a book, *The Man with a Shattered World* (1973). The narrative fragments have been joined together by Aleksandr Luria into a coherent narrative with a beginning, a middle, and an end. Luria's own comments explicate certain themes, comment on others, and above all add a medical context. Luria's textual parts are both explanative and supplementary. He not only explains Zasetsky's fragments and their meaning, but also introduces a medical and neurological context that make us as readers able to understand Zasetsky's narrative fragments as having been produced by a patient suffering from a certain type of brain trauma.

In his diaries Zasetsky repeatedly tried to account both for himself and others why he took great pains to write those entries. The point of his writing

> is to show how I have been, and still am, struggling to recover my memory. (. . .) I'd just sit trying to write this story, to dig up memories of my past that had vanished, to recall words and ideas that are as hard for me as ever. (. . .) By working on that one story of mine every day—even small amounts at a time—I hoped I'd be able to tell people about this illness and overcome it. (Luria, 1973, p. 84–85)

To Zasetsky the diary writing obviously was his attempt to tell a story piecing together his shattered experiences into something that at least had some resemblance to the world he once knew. Getting his world together has to do with his wish to be able to see himself as a person. He is trying to find who he is, and to find a connection between what happened to him during the war and who he is today. He seeks not only who he is, but also what he is. In this way Zasetsky's attempts to narrate is a sort of identity task; he tries to connect his present life with his previous life and his life to come. At the same time, he believes that his writing has a therapeutic effect; by writing he remembers and in that way he may vanquish his illness.

In his writings, Zasetsky has difficulties placing events in time and space—for instance, he preferred to express himself in an eternal presence. He also has problems connecting themes and events, resulting in a fragmentary text. In editing Zasetsky's text Aleksandr Luria attempts to place Zasetsky's fragments in time and space and to supply further biographical information, thus giving us a possibility to read, appreciate, and trust the narrative. By also adding medical comments—three lengthy "digressions" on brain anatomy and speech production—Luria further tries to explain, to give the reader an opportunity to understand the loss of normality, and hence to read the narrative. To Luria, Zasetsky is a patient whose special experience of the world he wants to convey and help the reader to understand and appreciate. Like his British-American colleague Oliver Sacks, Aleksandr Luria wants us as readers to understand that it is possible to perceive and understand in other ways than the ordinary.

In a way Luria's added comments are also a sort of narrative fragments that complement Zasetsky's own. Together with Luria's editorial work these two sets of fragments turn into a more or less coherent narrative. Luria's comments function as a sort of supportive or vicarious voice that fills out what he perceives is left out by Zasetsky. Without his vicarious, supplementary voice, we would probably never have been able to read Zasetsky's own narrative.

For instance, in order to create a narrative beginning, Aleksandr Luria prefaces the first excerpt from Zasetsky's diary by writing: "In the beginning it was all so simple. His past was much like other people's; life had its problems, but was simple enough, and the future seemed promising. Even now he loves to recall this, the pages of his diary reverting again and again to that lost life" (p. 3).

Luria creates a narrative frame that then is filled by the (lengthy) excerpts from Zasetsky's diary. In the same way, Luria ends the narrative and the book by adding a coda to the story:

"He continues to try to recover what was irretrievable, to make something comprehensible out of all the bits and pieces that remain of his life. He has returned to his story and is still working on it. It has no end" (p. 159).

In his comments Aleksandr Luria talks mainly about Zasetsky in the third person. Luria doesn't turn to Zasetsky in order to support him in the way Dorothy did in the example above. Rather, Luria turns to the reader and establishes a relationship with him or her, commenting on Zasetsky as a third person. Luria's voice supplements Zasetsky's, but at the same time it is pedagogic.

In summary, the bullet fragment that entered *his* brain had so devastated *his* world that *he* no longer had any sense of space, could not judge relationships between things, and perceived the world as broken into thousands of separate parts. As he put it, space "made no sense"; *he* feared it, for it lacked stability. (Luria, 1973, p. 61; italics added)

At the same time Luria's ambition is to show the world from the perspective of Zasetsky—how he experiences and literarily perceives the world. In Luria's textual comments we encounter Zasetsky's voice and perspective as an indirect voice. Luria analyzes Zasetsky's writing and rewrites his experience. Zasetsky's represented voice in Luria's textual comments has lost it narrative quality and instead turned into a report.

A central problem in the narrative text that Luria has produced is that Luria's vicarious and supplementary voice steps forward as the authoritative voice. We find the same phenomenon in Oliver Sacks's books about his patients; Oliver Sacks, like Aleksandr Luria, is the primary narrator entering into a relationship with the reader.

Consequently, Zasetsky's voice becomes subordinated to Luria's pedagogical medical voice that shows and explains. Zasetsky's attempts to formulate his own voice and identity become part of another narrative project and turns into a symptom. Zasetsky, like Sacks's patients, does not have any chance or ability to protest, defend himself, or formulate an alternative story—a counterstory.

At the same time there is something in Luria's text that makes it more complicated—a sincere ambition to heal a broken narrative. It is this sincerity that makes Luria's text into something else that is more than a medical text. What Luria attempts to do is to understand and reconstruct what we could call a lifeworld perspective on Zasetsky; it is the way Zasetsky experiences the world.

Substituting the teller: Carla's narrative

If you are not able to tell stories, to talk or even communicate, what about your identity? This is the problem that the American philosopher Hilde Lindemann Nelson writes about in an article about her sister Carla. Carla was born in the 1950s with hydrocephaly, something that not much could be done about at that time. As a consequence of this neural tube disorder her sister couldn't lift her head, grasp objects, or speak. Although Carla lived only 18 months, she was never able to express her own point of view, and even less able to tell about herself.

As a result her family engaged in what Hilde Lindemann Nelson calls the practice of holding the individual in personhood by constructing or maintaining a personal identity for her when she cannot, or can no longer, do it for herself (Lindemann Nelson, 2002, p. 30) .

By telling stories about Carla or telling stories that in some way included Carla, she became a part of the family. She also became part of a closely-knit web of stories that presented her as an agent or active subject. That is, as a child that preferred or liked certain things more than others, that had intentions and a will. Carla was treated as a person, with all the respect that is associated with having a personhood in our culture. Being a person means that other persons have certain moral obligations toward you, like taking care of you, comforting you, etc. You have to treat a person in certain ways, in contrast to your treatment of, for instance, nonliving things—something that is quite important if the person is not able to express his or her own point of view.

As readers we never get any examples of the stories that the family members told about Carla. We can find some examples in the research that David Goode reported on in his book *A World Without Words* (1995). In this book he discusses two girls, neither of whom could use language. Their families, however, are convinced that they can communicate with them in other ways. One of the things that the family members do is to create small stories about what the girls want. One of the girls is named Bianca. At one point during the fieldwork in the family Bianca became upset and started making sounds. Bianca's mother, Barbara, turned to David Goode, the researcher and offered an explanation, "She wants her milk." I asked her how she knew this, and she said that Bianca usually would have gotten her milk by now, but she (Barbara) had forgotten tonight (Goode, 1995, p.71).

This example is interesting because it illustrates how family members orient themselves toward the first person perspective of Bianca. They try to understand what she wants from her perspective. So even if Bianca's mother referred to her in the third person, she is invoking a first-person perspective; Bianca is treated as an agent although she can't communicative by language nor tell stories herself or about herself and her experiences.

The same appears to have happened in Carla's family. The individual family members tried to invoke Carla's first person perspective in at least some of the stories told about her.

By being the node of the family's narratives about her, Carla also received an identity—she became someone specific. Hilde Lindemann Nelson writes that the more stories about Carla the other five family members told, "the richer her [Carla's] identity became."

> Each of us in the family, I daresay, saw Carla in a slightly different light. Acting out of our various conceptions of who she was, we made a place for her among us, treating her according to how we saw her, and in so treating her, making her even more that person we saw.
>
> All of us, singly and severally, were contributing to what it meant to be Carla. To the extent that our narratives reflected faithfully who she was within our family (. . . .) The value of our narrative activity lay in the goodness of acknowledging a loved one's personhood with our own.

A central point that Hilde Lindemann Nelsons makes is that it is through telling stories about Carla her family members acknowledged her as a person, that is, treating Carla as if she is a person worthy of full respect. In order to be able to do this you have to acknowledge the possibility of Carla voicing a first-person perspective on herself, her family and the world.

Hence, in order to respect her person her narrative identity has to include a first-person perspective.

This was despite that fact that the stories that the family members told about Carla were all told entirely from the third-person perspective and also in the form of third person, that is, stories about another person where the teller is not identical to the main character of the story. This is substituting a narrative.

One problem with the idea of family members narrating Carla's identity is that they are telling stories about Carla that they don't know if she would accept or recognize as being true if she had had the capability to give voice to her own perspective. That is, Carla is positioned or narrated into an identity by others rather than positioning herself.

The story told by Hilde Lindemann Nelson is especially compelling because Carla was not able to present her own point of view. But situations where people are narratively positioned by others are quite common, as Hilde Lindemann Nelson has discussed elsewhere (Nelson, 2001). It is a common experience for most of us that other people tell stories about us and as a consequence position us a persons, assigning us an identity. If we don't accept the positioning or the story one possibility is of course to object to the story and try to revise it or complement it. If that doesn't work we have the further possibility of constructing and telling another story that we feel conveys our experiences and our perspective on events in a more accurate way. This new story told in critical dialogue with the first one is what Hilde Lindemann Nelson calls a counterstory (Nelson, 2001). To contest stories about oneself told by others, and maybe also tell counterstories, is probably a common experience in most families and in many other contexts.

In some contexts we have to fight for the right to tell our story and in that way sustain our sense of self. What we often want to do then is to tell a story from the first-person perspective, that is, telling something about our own experiences and history in order to tell about a defining moment— about how we came to be the persons we claim we are.

CONCLUSIONS

Telling autobiographical stories when you are narratively disabled, presupposes another person acting as your vicarious voice. This means that the relationship between the disabled person and the supporting person is of central interest. A central moral task seems to be to respect the disabled person's claim to personhood and not to reduce his or her life to stories that do not respect the claim of personhood.

Although all the vicarious tellers we have met tried in different ways to honor the disabled person's identity and sense of self, the tellers accomplished it in various ways.

Margret and Dorothy together tried to create order in the happenings that had so profoundly changed Dorothy's life. Basically the joint narrative was a result of a dialogue between Dorothy and Margret. It was a dialogue based on their longtime relationship, and on both their mutual explicit and implicit knowledge about each other.

Aleksandr Luria, as a medical doctor, tried to understand Zasetsky and make sense of his narratives, partly in a medical mode but also as told by a human being suffering from severe brain trauma. One further important task for Luria, informing his voice, was his relationship with the reader and his ambition to help the reader understand Zasetsky. As a consequence, Luria's vicarious voice in a sense incorporated Zasetsky's authorial and textual voice into his own, partly transforming it.

And finally, in Carla's case all family members constructed personal identities for Carla that in some way were part of their relationships to Carla as a person. The family members all subordinated their own vicarious voices to the potential (but never actualized) authorial voice of Carla.

A central problem is of course the risk that the authorial voice of the narratively disabled person disappears in the vicarious telling. As every narrative excludes other possible narratives, there is always a risk that other stories, construing the teller's identity differently, are never told. Having problems with using language more precisely also means having problems telling counternarratives or resisting the narratives told by the vicarious narrator.

Finally, the type of autobiographical narration we have met in this chapter challenges the individualistic assumptions of traditional autobiographical narration and identity. Traditionally autobiographical narration is based on an individual telling a first-person story about experiences that he or she "owns." Furthermore, the individual's identity is constituted through this type of narration.

This is obviously an idea that becomes problematic with respect to persons who suffer from a severe disease like Alzheimer's or are aphasic due to brain trauma. In most cases the individual is unable to use language in ordinary ways and as a consequence will have severe problems telling stories about his/her past and constructing autobiographical narratives, an identity, and a sense of self.

Traditionally a person is capable of narrating him/herself and as a consequence of establishing himself or herself as responsible for both the telling as an act and the told life. The cases discussed in this chapter put a question mark around these ideas of responsibility. Carla had severe problems with both these aspects, while Zasetsky and Dorothy to various degrees were able to tell, maintain, and claim responsibility for their stories and lives. In all cases they had to share responsibility with another person, which shifts some of the responsibility over to the supporting person.

This can possibly impel us to be careful with the idea of using the individual and his or her autobiographical narration as the paradigmatic case for autobiographical narration. Perhaps we should instead consider the autobiographical narration as something that is created together with others, which introduces the concept of different voices. As I have tried to show here, this is a situation that is driven to its extreme when one of the individuals has serious communicative functional hinderances.

ACKNOWLEDGMENT

The study was supported by a grant from Swedish Council for Working Life and Social Research.

REFERENCES

Antelius, E. (2007). The meaning of the present: Hope and foreclosure in narrations about people with severe brain damage. *Medical Anthropology Quarterly, 21,* 324–342.

Bakhtin, M. (1984). *Problems of Dostoevsky's poetics.* Minneapolis, MN: University of Minnesota Press.

Brockmeier, J. (2008) Language, experience, and the "traumatic gap": How to talk about 9/11? In Hydén, L.-C. & Brockmeier, J., (Eds.), *Health, illness and culture: Broken narratives* (pp. 16–35). New York: Routledge.

Brockmeier, J., & Carbaugh, D. (2001). Introduction. In J. Brockmeier & D. Carbaugh (Eds.) *Narrative and identity: Studies in autobiography, self and culture* (pp. 1–22). Amsterdam: John Benjamins.

Bruner, J. (2001). Self-making and world-making. In J. Brockmeier & D. Carbaugh (Eds.) *Narrative and identity: Studies in autobiography, self and culture* (pp. 25–38). Amsterdam: John Benjamins.

Cicourel, A. V. (1975). Discourse and text: Cognitive and linguistic processes in studies of social structure. *Versus, 12,* 33–83.

Eakin, P. J. (2001). Breaking rules: the consequences of self-narrations. *Biography. 24,* 113–127.

Fivush, R. (1994). Constructing narrative, emotion, and self in parent–child conversations about the past. In U. Neisser & R. Fivush (Eds.), *The remembering self: Construction and accuracy in the self-narrative* (pp. 136–157). New York: Cambridge University Press.

Goffman, E. (1981). *Forms of talk.* Philadelphia: University of Pennsylvania Press.

Goldstein, K. (1948). *Language and language disturbances. Aphasic symptom complexes and their significance for medicine and theory of language.* New York: Grune and Stratton.

Goode, D. (1995). *A world without words. The social construction of children born deaf and blind.* Philadelphia: Temple University Press.

Gusdorf, G. (1980). Conditions and limits of autobiography. In J. Olney (Ed.), *Autobiography: Essays theoretical and critical* (pp. 28–48). Princeton, NJ: Princeton University Press.

Hydén, L. C. (1995). The rhetoric of recovery and change. *Culture, Medicine, and Psychiatry, 19,* 73–90.

Josselson, R. (2004). On becoming the narrator of one's own life. In A. Lieblich, D. McAdams, & R. Josselson (Eds.), *Healing plots: The narrative basis of psychotherapy* (pp. 111–127). Washington, DC: American Psychological Association.

Labov, W. (1972). The transformation of experience in narrative syntax. In W. Labov (Ed.), *Language in the inner city* (pp. 354–405). Philadelphia: University of Pennsylvania Press.

Luria, A. R. (1973). *The man with a shattered world.* New York: Basic Books.

Medved, M. & Brockmeier, J. (2008). Talking About the unthinkable: Neurotrauma and the "catastrophic reaction." In Hydén, L.-C. & Brockmeier, J., (Eds.), *Health, illness and culture: Broken narratives* (pp. 54–72). New York: Routledge.

Miller, P. J. (1994). Narrative practices: Their role in socialization and self-construction. In U. Neisser & R. Fivush (Eds.), *The remembering self: Construction and accuracy in the self-narrative* (pp. 158–179). New York: Cambridge University Press.

Mishler, E. G. (1984). *The discourse of medicine. Dialectics of medical interviews.* Norwood, NJ: Ablex Publishing Company.

Nelson, H. L. (2001). *Damaged identities, narrative repair.* Ithaca, NY: Cornell University Press.

Nelson, H. L. (2002). What child is this? *Hastings Center Report, 32,* 29–38.

Ochs, E., & Capps, L. (2001). *Living narrative: Creating lives in everyday story-telling.* Cambridge, MA: Harvard University Press.

Örulv, L., & Hydén, L.-C. (2006). Confabulation: Sense-making, self-making and world-making in dementia. *Discourse Studies, 8,* 677–703.

Sabat, S. R. (2001). *Experience of Alzheimer's disease. Life through a tangled veil.* Oxford, UK: Blackwell.

Sacks, O. (1985). *The man who mistook his wife for a hat.* London: Duckworth.

Schechtman, M. (1996). *The constitution of selves.* Ithaca, NY: Cornell University Press.

Vygotsky, L. S. (1987). Thinking and speech. In *The collected works of L. S. Vygotsky,* Vol. 1 (pp. 39–285). New York: Kluwer Academic.

Weintraub, K. J. (1978). *The value of the individual: Self and circumstance in autobiography.* Chicago: Chicago University Press.

Young, K., & Saver, J. L. (2001). The neurology of narrative. *Substance: A review of theory and literary criticism, 30*(1/2), 72–84.

4 Talking About the Unthinkable
Neurotrauma and the "Catastrophic Reaction"

Maria I. Medved and Jens Brockmeier

For most people, the experience of a serious and unexpected disease or injury is catastrophic. Sudden sickness or disability usually comes with fundamental changes, throwing one into a new and unknown reality. The experience of living in this overwhelming new reality often leads to an existential crisis; all of a sudden former ways of understanding one's self and the world are no longer adequate, but new ways seem impossible to come by.

As has often been reported, narrativization of this crisis is a crucial way in which people attempt to understand and possibly come to terms with it. In this process, narrative, as well as the entire discursive and social context in which it takes place becomes indistinguishable from the very experience of illness. In the act of telling, meaning construction or "acts of meaning" (Bruner, 1990) take place that offer the ill the possibility of coping with their shaken sense of self and being in the world.

Many studies exploring the process of narrative meaning-making after illness have shown the high degree of reflexivity and cognitive sophistication it entails. The underlying assumption of most of these studies has been that the disease or injury does not influence the sufferer's essential ability to narrate. But what about individuals whose fundamental linguistic and cognitive capability to narrate itself is affected from neurological lesions (whether due to an accident, stroke, or neurodegenerative disorder)? If disease or injury is experienced as a catastrophic event in and of itself, and narrative is used to cope with such an event, then damage to the linguistic and cognitive abilities required for narrative must be perceived as especially catastrophic.

The neurologist Kurt Goldstein was particularly interested in this sort of psychological catastrophe. Although he did not specifically study illness narratives, he did examine how neurologically-impaired people attempted to come to terms with their, as it were, twofold disaster. According to Goldstein, problematic adaptation to the changed self after neurotrauma might result in what he called a "catastrophic reaction." Our purpose is to take a closer look at what he meant by such a catastrophic reaction, exploring how it can enrich our present understanding of the broken narratives of people who suffer from serious brain injuries.

Kurt Goldstein (1878–1965), as Oliver Sacks (1995) describes, is one of the most important, contradictory, and forgotten figures in neurology. In fact, if someone comes across Goldstein's work, and this might happen, Sacks suggests, mostly coincidently, it can turn into a real discovery, an intellectual surprise. As happened to us. Our own introduction to Goldstein's work occurred when we were trying to gain a better understanding of how people with neurological damage come to terms with both their new lives and their "new" brains. Developing such a comprehensive understanding requires a broader and more holistic view than is offered by traditional neurophysiology or neuroscience. It needs a neuro*psychological* vision, the vision of a *person* in his or her being in the world.

This vision is precisely what we found in Goldstein's work. Compared to most traditional neurological literature focusing on isolating lesions and deficit measurement, Goldstein's work offers a differentiated and sensitive approach, one that focuses on the living reality of human subjectivity. Even the titles of his works reflect this focus, as in the article *The effect of brain damage on the personality* (Goldstein, 1952). While things might be different for laboratory neuroscientists, for anyone concerned with the understanding and rehabilitation of people, both human subjectivity and human agency must be central to the issue of neurotrauma.

Throughout much of his research Goldstein points out that the thoughts, emotions, and behaviors of neurological patients are produced not only by their brains, but also by their experiences in particular social environments. In this view, the mind not only has a neuronal existence, but also a cultural existence. Upon closer examination, even basic reflexes such as the knee jerk prove to be not so physiologically "basic" as they might initially seem. Rather, Goldstein holds, they can vary according to both the organism's state and the specific environmental conditions. Many of his insights were gained in the first decades of the last century, among others, when, during World War I, Goldstein was director of the Military Hospital for Brain-Injured Soldiers, an experience that resulted in his 1942 book, *Aftereffects of Brain Injuries in War*. After the war, he continued his research as professor of neurology and psychiatry at the University of Berlin, and as director of various clinics in Berlin and Frankfurt, before, as a Jew, he left Germany in the 1930s and immigrated to the United States.

Today, some of Goldstein's arguments may seem unusual. While one reason for this might be his dated terminology, this is also because his overall approach to human reality was holistic. Combining neurological dimensions with psychological dimensions of human experience, his views starkly contrast the biological emphasis of contemporary medicine. Here is someone who views symptoms as attempted solutions, locates cognition across multiple minds, and suggests that individuality does not involve one, but multiple "creatures." Clearly, his central ideas have continued to remain as unusual and as radical.

In this chapter, we draw on Goldstein's contribution to the understanding of people's reactions to neurological lesions, and more specifically on the "catastrophic reaction." We begin with a reading of Goldstein's main ideas relating to the catastrophic reaction, as developed in his book *The Organism*. Goldstein introduced the term catastrophic reaction in order to describe problematic psychological adjustment to cognitive impairment. Specifically, he notes, catastrophic reactions result from a blend of extreme confusion, shock, and intense anxiety. Such a state appears when the organism experiences a trauma and continues trying to do new things in old ways. Inevitably, the "impossibility to do so leads to continued unrest [and] to catastrophic reactions" (Goldstein, 1934/1995, p. 193).

Goldstein divided behavior into two classes: ordered and disordered. Actions that are adequate for the demands of the situation may be considered as ordered behavior. Ordered behavior usually engenders the person to experience his own behavior as adequate and consistent, and this consistency is typically accompanied by a feeling of calmness. On the other hand, when the demands of the situation are beyond a person's capacity, disordered behavior may result, and the person will experience his own behavior as inconsistent, which is typically accompanied by anxiety. The latter is often the case with individuals suffering from brain injury, who often find themselves behaving in a disordered fashion because their neuropsychological "performance capacity [is] disproportionate" to the demands of their environment (Goldstein, 1934/1995).

Another important concept Goldstein uses is that of "abstract attitude." Abstract attitude refers to an individual's ability to both think imaginatively and move beyond the "mindless concrete." In Goldstein's era, this concept was sometimes referred to as "symbolic expression" (Henry Head) or "representational function" (Willem von Woerkom). Without abstract attitude, a person's ability to make sense of the anxiety that accompanies a disordered state is severely reduced. Goldstein notes that this is because, without abstract attitude, it is difficult for the individual to "become conscious of [one]self" (1934/1995, p. 232). As a consequence, there is a qualitative shift in the individual's experience of his own anxiety in that the person does not have the feeling of anxiety, but due to the lack of abstract attitude, *is* the anxiety.

For individuals with brain injury, many areas of life become challenging. In many cases, even simple and familiar tasks are no longer easily accomplished, often leading to a fairly continuous onslaught of intense anxiety. Ultimately, this culminates in a catastrophic reaction. In Goldstein's words, catastrophic reactions are

> not only "inadequate" but also disordered, inconstant, inconsistent, and embedded in physical and mental shock. In these situations, the individual feels himself unfree, buffeted, and vacillating. He experiences a shock affecting not only his own person, but the surrounding world as well. (1934/1995, p. 49)

What a person experiences in such a moment is the "breaking down or dissolution of the world and a shattering of his own self" (p. 232). To be sure, individuals do whatever they can to avoid the horrifying disequilibrium of a catastrophic reaction. Goldstein identifies two ways in which people with brain damage (and in fact, *all* people) can cope and reduce the descent into a catastrophic reaction. The first way is for the individual to "shrink" or reduce the environmental demands. In this case the individual "clings tenaciously to the order that is adequate for him but that appears abnormally primitive, rigid, and compulsive" (p. 54) in order to avoid the anxiety associated with disordered behavior; for example, sticking to routines and ignoring difficult situations that require new behaviors can accomplish this. The second way is to latch onto something concrete such as objects in one's environment. This is because without abstract attitude, it is impossible to use generic concepts, ideas, plans, or goals to guide one's self. Here, tangible objects are needed in place of abstract thought in order to assist the individual with "centering" or grounding himself. Thus, individuals cling "to something 'filled,' to an object to which they can react or with which they can establish contact through activity" (p. 55). Without concrete reference points, there is an increased likelihood of disordered behavior and along with it the increased risk of being driven into a catastrophic reaction.

Using Goldstein's neuropsychological interpretation of catastrophic reaction as a general framework, we now will explore how the study of narrative can help us better understand the dynamics involved in such a reaction. In particular, we will look at how neurocognitive changes hinder one's capacity to use narrative as a mode of thought instrumental to comprehending what has happened. We will point out that the breakdown of narrative's main cognitive and discursive functions allow us to catch a glimpse in the inner workings of what Goldstein called a catastrophic reaction. Some of the core functions of narrative relevant here are the creation of coherence, distancing from events, binding others into communication, evaluation of experiences, and exploration of alternative possibilities ("possible worlds"). We have described these functions in more detail elsewhere (Medved & Brockmeier, 2004). So to begin our examination and discussion of these functions against the backdrop of Goldstein's thoughts, we open with a case study.

We draw on an interview with Ms. E. We selected Ms. E's interview from a corpus of interviews because it demonstrates what we think is an exemplary "narrative breakdown," reflecting Goldstein's notion of catastrophic reaction. As we will see in a moment, Ms. E appears to be in the midst of the process of becoming aware of her precariously changed state of mind as she is faced with her own new limits to comprehend her new life and self.

The interview took place nine weeks after Ms. E was admitted to hospital for an aneurysm (a ballooning and eventual rupturing of a blood vessel) of her right anterior communicating artery (AcoA). This artery has many branches perfusing numerous structures including the frontal lobes. At the time of the interview, Ms. E displayed symptoms of what neuropsychologists refer to as "AcoA syndrome," which is a mixture of amnesia, confabulation, and personality change (for a full list of symptoms, see DeLuca & Diamond, 1995). Although her scores on a measure of gross cognitive dysfunction placed her as performing in the "normal range," she experienced particular difficulty with tasks involving abstract conceptualization and memory.

However, this is only the medical picture. While it provides information about Ms. E's neurocognitive functioning, it does not tell us much about her as a person. So who is she? Ms. E is in her mid-40s and lives with her husband and primary-school aged daughter. For most of her professional life she has pursued a career in insurance sales, working her way up from salesperson to regional manager, a career trajectory of which she is proud. Like many women, she views herself as someone struggling to balance family and career, but appeared to be satisfied with her standing in both domains. Disciplined, well groomed, cheerful, and enjoying an active social life—that is what Ms. E must have been before her stroke radically changed it all.

And then? Let us present one uninterrupted excerpt taken from our interview with her. We think this extended excerpt of what, in fact, often was more a conversation, captures the particular narrative flow of her discourse better than any segments artificially separated for presentation. Granted, no interview or conversation, however extended, can possibly capture the developmental trajectory leading to a catastrophic reaction; the "reaction" started before we met Ms. E and will continue afterwards. Nor can the excerpt fully capture the emotional turmoil, the sheer physicality of the existential drama that we see unfolding: her agitated and repetitive hand gestures, her furrowed brow and pursed mouth, and the hectic prosody and the explosive sound of her speech.

The excerpt starts with Ms. E describing her weekend.

Interviewer (I): Tell me, did you go out on a weekend pass last weekend?

Ms. E (E): Yeah.

I: How did that work out?

E: Not very well.

I: What happened?

E: Well, again, *MY* husband married someone who *pays* the bills, *cleans* the house, *takes* care of Jenny, *makes* the meals, like you *know,* I'm superwoman. {shrugs}

I: Yes . . .

E: A(:)nyway, so he asked me "*Are you* going to do the groceries" "NO(:)" "Why not?" >"Because I don't feel up to it.< *I'll* make a list, we can make together and you can go. It won't *kill* you to go to the grocery store."

I: And this happened last weekend?

E: Yeah. And the(:)n my mother arrived. My mother and my brother and a sister arrived from Alberta. My godmother, her son and her daughter, came up from Maryland, so *you got* to entertain. >They're only here for a weekend.< You know so(:) that was stressful.

I: Yeah. Well that would be stressful considering that you were just in the hospital.

E: I like to entertain, like (.) and we bought another house, this would be our un, deux, trois, quatre, *fourth* house and we discovered that there were things that weren't the way they were supposed to be and we were supposed to be closing at the end of the April. >So we were saying we don't want, *you* know we don't know (.) if we want to close, we don't know if we want to go through until we see the house and appraiser < and he said like, "*who are you?*" and I said I'M A REAL ESTATE REP. I WANT to ask you a few things and I AM going to avoid problems if I could.

I: So this was on the weekend?

E: Yeah.

I: My gosh, that *was* a busy weekend.

E: Oh yeah.

I: Gosh

E: A(:)nd . . . what else was there? Oh yeah, May's birthday, my niece and Godchild. My brother in Brandenberg, her son, it was his birthday last weekend and we were *trying* to figure out how to arrange, I mean he's going to be 11.

I: Hmm. Obviously very busy. Uh, how is it? Is there anything that you, yourself, feel that you've lost any memories or has your thinking changed in any way?

E: Yes.

I: Can you tell me a bit about that?

E: Like today, there was supposed to be a big meeting in what I call the gym. The auditorium, some people call it the cafeteria. *Big meeting*, like full gym.

I: What about?

E: Um, the benefits that the hospital has and *I* am one of the hospital's benefits. YOU can buy your home insurance at a reduced rate and pay it from here. So they want it, I'll sign people with the hospital and so on. And so, I had it organized, I had it organized like a month ahead. When you go they said, OK, April this and this and I write it down and I had all my schedule in, put in place and all of a sudden, I'm in this hospital. I was told ok, "Will you go if you can come and go as you please and at your work too?" and I said, "ah, yes." I can't take two or three weeks off my job. I'M A SALES REP. I have a mortgage to pay, I have a daughter to raise, you know what I mean? I won't do that. I don't think I need to. And the fella that I was with at work says "I agree with you," until I came here and they started testing me and I'm going "OH my God."

I: What do you mean?

E: I don't feel there is anything wrong with me until something hits me in the face and I'm like "Oh MY God." (.) Like the reason this person is here [assessing me] was because I do not remember it at all.

I: Does that happen to you often?

E: Oh, often.

I: Can you give an example?

E: Well(:), I was sitting here and someone said to me "Do you know where you are now?" And *I* have worked as a volunteer in this hospital for 5 years . . .

What happens here can be described in neuropsychological terms as a catastrophic reaction as well as in narrative terms as a narrative breakdown. Our analysis incorporates both perspectives, linking Goldstein's perspective with a narrative-analytical perspective. In certain respects, a similar effort of combining neurological and narrative perspectives has been made by Young and Saver (2001), who distinguish between four types of neurologically-induced "dysnarration." One type, the type apparently represented by Ms. E's discourse, called "unbound narration," is typically associated with damage to frontal lobe structures. This type of dysnarration occurs when individuals are unable to self-monitor and, as a result, tell stories unconstrained by actual memories and experiences. In our analysis, we would like to qualify, and expand on, this description of unbound narration by identifying several narrative functions. In the case of Ms. E, her narratives serve (or are supposed to serve) all of these different functions. As already mentioned, we refer to them as coherence, distancing, evaluative, communicative, and explorative functions. Although we present and discuss them separately, they are, of course, intimately intertwined.

COHERENCE FUNCTIONING

One general function of narrative is that it offers cognitive and communicative coherence; it creates a synthesis of the world. Narrative synthesizes personal experiences and sensations that may otherwise be disconnected and random. The coherence of such a narrative synthesis can be based on a variety of criteria that encompasses thematic (what the story is about), spatial (what happens at a particular location), temporal (what happens in a particular sequence), to historical (what happens at a particular time) aspects. There are also compositional features such as genres, narrative models, and perspectives or points of view that can make a story coherent. Furthermore, there are rhetorical and stylistic qualities (metaphors, metonymies, parables and other figures of speech) contributing to the coherence of a narrative (Brockmeier, 2004). Paul Ricoeur (1991) has argued that the basis for this coherence is narrative "configuration" or "emplotment," which is an act of integration that transforms various incidents into a whole. In essence, it helps the individual to form "a synthesis out of heterogeneous elements" (p. 21). For many of us, talking about events and emotions and organizing them into a well-formed narrative plot can be a struggle even under normal conditions. However, in cases of illness or disability the struggle for well-formed narratives is intensified, particularly when coupled with serious neurocognitive difficulties. Such is the case with Ms. E.

In the wake of the neurocognitive limitations brought on by her stroke, Ms. E frequently grapples with assembling a coherent narrative. In the interview, a discernable emplotment does not seem to emerge regardless of what criteria we apply: thematic, temporal, spatial, historical, compositional, or otherwise. Her narrative is like a raging river sucking up everything in its path; a stream of consciousness out of control. Not only is there a mix of memories of real events with fictive events, but also blends of unrelated linguistic associations (e.g., pseudonyms for the word "gym"), clichés and stock phrases (e.g., "you can buy your home insurance at a reduced rate"), and fragments from scripts of everyday life, both real and imaginative (e.g., "we bought another house . . ."). Interspersed throughout her thoughts are moments of doubt and glimpses of the present (e.g., "I do not remember it at all").

Interestingly, Ms. E's lack of coherence occurs between what appears to be distinct experiences or episodes as well as within what appears to be the same experiences or episodes (e.g., in "I like to entertain, like we bought another house"). In the example of buying a new house, one might be tempted to make the connection that perhaps Ms. E wanted a bigger living room to entertain, thus suggesting a kind of hidden but identifiable coherence to this part of the story. What helps in most conversations that seem incoherent is to ask the speaker what was intended. This, however, is to no avail. When Ms. E is asked, for example, whether she feels as if she has lost any memories or whether her thinking has changed, she mentions a "big meeting" in the gym, a response that seemingly has no connection to the original question. That there is no beginning or end to her narrative flow and that there are none of the self-referential markers we often encounter in conversations (i.e., I experienced this, I just read this in the paper, I've always had this wish, etc.) does not help to clarify the relations between the storyteller and the listener.

Another criterion of coherence that might be appropriate for understanding Ms. E's talk is the emotional tenor or drive of her narrative. One might argue that Ms. E's stories demonstrate a particular kind of emotional or affective coherence. But if they have a connecting emotional core organized around her anxiety and angst, this emotional "coherence" is perceived and attributed from the outside. It does not help Ms. E herself to organize her talk, and in particular, it does not appear to help her make sense of her situation or of her endless stream of stories. Nor does it help her to communicate this sense, and thus, to connect to someone else. To be sure, this sense of being permanently out of control distresses her even more as her damaged brain is continuously burdened with a relentless flow of information and associations. In sum, Ms. E is in a permanent state of extreme cognitive and emotional stress and, at the same time, experiences complete helplessness—a veritable quagmire she cannot escape.

Oddly enough, the endless flow of details that contributes to this critical state may also help her cope. As Goldstein observed, one way people react when losing their grip on their ability to reflect on the unthinkable is to cling to the tangible, to something firm. If this is the case, it could be that Ms. E's apparently uncontrolled stream of concrete details were simultaneously steadying her, giving her something stable to hold onto.

DISTANCING FUNCTIONING

Following Goldstein's discussion of the tangible we will now introduce the distancing function of narrative. One of the prominent qualities of narrative discourse is that it renders the immediate and fleeting qualities of an experience into an "external object." This process entails transforming our perceptions, thoughts, and emotions into a unitary and meaningful structure, something that can then be kept at bay, considered, and reflected on. While this is likely to be true for all language, narrative, in particular, affords us the capacity to construe extended complex meaning structures from fleeting experiences. As Bruner notes,

> we distance ourselves from the immediacy of events by converting what we've encountered into story form. We give that story form a standing on its own, regardless of who's telling it, in what setting, with what ends in mind. Our master interpretants for assigning meanings to what is said, read, or encountered, unless again there are indications to the contrary, are narrative or script-like in nature. We render the bare-bones of the encounter into the constituents of narrative. (2002, p. 89)

But what happens to someone's ability to defend themselves against the unstructured vagrancies of life when their capability to narrate and thus create distance from the chaotic here and now has gone askew? Obviously Ms. E's options to cope with the onslaught of "cognitive stimuli," to couch it in a clinical language, as well as with the intense feelings or "emotional stimuli" that overcome her after her stroke are dramatically reduced. As we have seen, she has to contend with a relentless flux of memories, associations, phrases, clichés, and scripted stories, a flux that is not stabilized or slowed by her brief moments of distance or self-observation. The point we want to highlight now is that she is virtually caught in a temporal immediacy that precludes any kind of self-distance and reflexivity. When Ms. E questions whether she had a neuropsychological assessment ("because I don't remember at all"), she seems to be struggling to sustain the distance needed to further develop this memory into a more extended thought. In this particular case, despite succeeding to hold on to this memory for a moment, all she eventually manages is to express the horror of it all ("Oh my God"). While interviewing Ms. E we had the impression that her experience of her mental and emotional life felt like waves of an indecipherable flood constantly threatening to overwhelm her—so much so that this sense eventually came to dominate her entire world and self.

This experience of intense anxiety and panic is similar to what happens to people suffering from posttraumatic stress disorder. In cases of posttraumatic stress disorder, the impact of the traumatic event can be so catastrophic that it paralyzes the power of narrative to shelter the individual from the volatile and intense emotions associated with the trauma. Thus, in the case of Ms. E, what overwhelms her is a combination of two catastrophic experiences: the trauma of her stroke and the trauma of her narrative breakdown.

While we interpret Ms. E's broken narratives in terms of a lack of narrative distancing, Goldstein would probably frame it in terms of abstract attitude. As previously mentioned, without abstract attitude the individual is unable to move beyond the concreteness of immediate experience. We believe this view overlaps with the narrative perspective in the sense that distancing also requires the creation of an abstract attitude. Taking Bruner's narrative distancing one step further, we might call this "narrative abstraction," as it refers to the inherent quality of narrative to create cognitive and emotional distance to keep a troubling experience or thought at arm's length.

COMMUNICATIVE FUNCTIONING

The communicative function of narrative is to connect the teller to the listener and the listener to the teller. This connection unfolds when both the teller and the listener are intersubjectively engaged, constituting what in narrative theory is called a "narrative event," in contrast with the content being told, the "narrated event." Typically, the teller initiates the story with the goal of involving his or her listener, who, in turn, commits him- or herself to the telling. In other words, the ideal listener will listen attentively, comment, and provide additional details, ironic variations, criticism, or even counternarratives. In doing so, listeners can legitimate, alter, challenge, or silence the initiated story. For these reasons, many researchers argue that narratives are essentially coconstructed; they are communicative events, sites of intense intersubjective exchange.

Ms. E's narratives are certainly communicative events. Throughout our meetings she appeared to enjoy sharing her stories and we always encountered a social and inviting person. However, Ms. E also engaged in extended monologues and although she would stop if questioned, her answers often lacked conversational fine-tuning. A major difficulty, on a rudimentary level, was that in the face of Ms. E's pressured stream of narrative there was simply very little conversational space. Most of her stories were not tailored for a listening audience; there was not much monitoring for intelligibility, nor did she attend to the effect her stories were having on the listener. Ms. E appeared to be talking at, rather than with, the listener, and sometimes her narratives resembled a form of inner speech. This is not to say all her stories were communicatively unsuccessful; some were extremely poignant and drew the listener in. But this binding, in general, was short-lived.

Still, there is the impression of a strong communicative interest, a wish to reach out, an effort to connect, even if it seemed impeded. How can we understand this restriction? Again returning to Goldstein's framework, this restriction results from the absence of abstract attitude. Without distancing from the immediacy of one's psychological life, it is difficult to connect to someone else, the listener, who lives beyond this immediacy. Without this dialogical dimension of narrative, the teller wavers between communicative intention and failure. As a consequence, social contacts become impoverished and it is impossible to utilize the abstract attitude of someone else, that is, the understanding, empathy, and help of someone else in order to coconstruct one's own narratives, narratives that could bring structure and wholeness to one's shattered world.

As Goldstein points out, there are many situations where individuals who lack abstract attitude benefit from "shared cognition." Young children who do not have abstract attitude, are able to live and develop primarily because they are able to socially relate to, as well as rely on, people who organize their world in a way which exposes them to demands that are appropriate to their ability. The profound social nature of children enables them to live in what Lev Vygotsky, Goldstein's contemporary, called a "zone of proximal development" (1930/1978). As Vygotsky and Luria (1930/1994) emphasized, the more the abstract attitude of an individual (which is mediated by signs and, especially, language) is limited, the more social interaction with others takes on importance. Joint discursive activity such as narrative coconstruction, which sometime embraces performative modes (Brockmeier, 2005), can also support narrative functions such as the creation of coherence and distancing, even if a person lacks abstract attitude. One of Ms. E's recurring difficulties is that she "ignores" the efforts of others to discursively "offer" her the narrative resources and the abstract attitude she lacks. Relating this back to Ms. E's everyday life, listeners may eventually "overwrite" her talk and story altogether, a process described by Lars-Christer Hydén (2008).

EVALUATIVE FUNCTIONING

Narrative is not limited to creating coherence, giving distance to experiences, emotions, and thoughts, and communicating events and ideas; it also takes an evaluative stance. It articulates values, and positions the narrator towards the narrated event as well as within the narrative event. Storytelling is more than just an act of conveying information, content, and plot; it is a practice that frames, even if not necessarily consciously, events, experiences, and ideas to fit a particular evaluative matrix, a matrix that includes the teller, the listener, and the rest of the world. Narrative takes a stance and offers a perspective on both what is said and not said. In this section, we will concentrate on Ms. E's stance towards herself and, implicitly, towards others.

As we have previously noted, Ms. E's stories sometimes appear rigid and scripted, told in a rote, nonspontaneous manner. Furthermore, the fragments of content and plot as well as the explicit evaluative stance appear standardized, as when she quotes slogans and stock phrases. One has the impression that most of her broken narratives seem to have been told many times before and that she seems to be drawing from a reserve of well-rehearsed memories readily accessible even in her time of crisis.

Oddly enough, in these story fragments, Ms. E consistently positions herself as being in control of her life, and judging from how she presents herself in her memories, she probably once was; for example, during episodes in which she insists on a full assessment of a new house or that her husband do the shopping. In any case she is in charge. She presents herself as a woman who knows what needs to be done and goes about directing others on what needs doing.

Interestingly, Ms. E's fixed evaluative stance is not confined to premorbid memories; it also emerges in postmorbid memories. It seems these "new" memories have also been incorporated into her narratives. Consider Ms. E's experience of being in the hospital. To continue her self-positioning as a woman in charge, she needs to develop a suitable story that explains why she is in a hospital. As we see, her story reveals that she is doing volunteer work.

Notice that this construal needs to be forced to fit her evaluative stance because her stories may not mirror her actual situation very well. Even Ms. E, in her present situation, is aware that a volunteer in a hospital does not have to stay there 24 hours per day. In order to make her story convincing she puts in as much effort as possible to turn it into a narrative performance, performing in a breathless manner. On the one hand, we believe this effort is due to a felt need to make her story persuasive, so to avoid any space for skepticism. On the other hand, we also understand her evaluative attitude as part of this predicament. The tenor of her narratives is that things are under her control, and that nothing in her life has changed. Thus, there is no need, nor possibility, to take action or deal with her posttraumatic situation. Her stories are not only incongruent with her present everyday life, but also with her turbulent affective life. While she positions herself as in control, she is highly anxious and agitated. And if this were not enough, the continuous experience of this inconsistency further deepens her inner panic towards a catastrophic reaction.

Why, then, does Ms. E continue to position herself as being in control? Why does she insist on claiming her life has not really changed after her stroke? And why does she continue to tell stories from a parallel world, the world of her former life. One reason could be psychological: Her normalizing and reassuring evaluative stance is directed not only to the external addressee, but also toward the teller—herself. In a situation where her experience of the world she knew has gone awry, Ms. E desperately attempts to convince herself that she is on top of her game. Even when she momentarily appears to admit that this might not be entirely true (when "something hits [her] in the face," or she doesn't "feel up to" shopping or other important activities), she implies that of course she would be able to do them if she chose.

A second reason why she continues her self-positioning attitude is neurological: Nuanced evaluative functioning requires a kind of cognitive flexibility and reflexivity that is similar to Goldstein's abstract attitude.

As these abilities are seriously affected by her stroke, Ms. E's narratives remain "stuck" without any chance of alternative plotting. Still, we believe it is important to be aware of the ambivalent nature of this stance. From Goldstein's point of view, Ms. E's rigid evaluative stance could be seen as a way of coping, as he argued that individuals with neurotrauma often reduce their world in order to simplify it. In this way, they at least have a chance to engage in ordered behavior. In the case of Ms. E, her narratives likely serve this same purpose.

EXPLORATIVE FUNCTIONING

One of the most powerful and creative qualities of narrative is its explorative function. Narrative allows us to explore two sides of human experience: the real and the possible. It allows us to speculate about what might have been, what is, and what might continue to be. These excursions into the possible and subjunctive are central to our narrative imagination. They open up alternative visions of life and offer various perspectives of our possible lives and worlds (Brockmeier, 2002). In short, the explorative function of narrative is about probing and extending the horizon of human possibilities.

Although an explorative attitude might be said to be inherent to all narrative discourse, in the stories of Ms. E, it was difficult to discern an effort to take advantage of the explorative potentials of narrative. For instance, she rarely took us up on offers to engage on the subjunctive dimensions of her life, such as in anticipating a possible future for herself. We were strangely touched when we noticed her resistance to delve into "how things could be" or "could possibly become." Perhaps she could not anticipate a new life, or did not want to, for she was fully absorbed in already living a new life, as unwelcome as it was. We often had the impression that all of her narrative resources were taken up by the current crisis, leaving no cognitive or emotional space to imagine life alternatives, realistic or fictitious.

Still, one might be tempted to read Ms. E's announcements such as that she is "one of the hospital's benefits" as evidence of the explorative function. One might want to understand them as outlooks into a different world, as indicators that she is trying to evoke a counterreality in which she can continue to live in a "normalized" story world where she is an agent that is in control rather than a patient who is out of control. However, after talking with her for extended periods we have come to see utterances like this as being more indicative of the "normalizing" evaluative functioning of her discourse. In principle, Ms. E's narratives might be capable of fulfilling exploratory functions. However, we did not recognize any evidence of imaginative attempts; it was as if everything was swallowed up by the here and now. Had we a chance to ask Professor Goldstein, he would likely have pointed out that exploration of alternative lives and futures would hardly be possible for someone like Ms. E. because exploration of this kind requires abstract attitude.

A WORLD IN FLUX

So far, we have studied the workings, or perhaps more accurately, the failure of the workings of narrative in a Goldsteinian catastrophic reaction. We have also demonstrated how taking a closer look at narrative and its functioning can be a particularly fruitful way to further our understanding of such a catastrophic reaction. In recent literature, there is increasing support for the suggestion that narrativizing traumatic experience of injury or disease is crucial to comprehending, and ultimately, coming to terms with trauma. Yet, as we noted, the experiences of those with a damaged brain are chaotic, unique, and all but easy to plot in a storyline. Is there really a storyline to figure out what is going on with a brain that is suddenly, radically, and, likely, permanently transmogrified?

In examining an interview sequence with a woman suffering from the consequences of a stroke we have attempted to explore why the narrativization of a cerebral damage experience is particularly difficult. What makes this experience so precarious is that it involves the actual breakdown of the capacity of narrating or, at least, a far-reaching reduction of some of narrative's main functions. Investigating the coherence, evaluative, communicative, distancing, and explorative functions, we saw that all of them were affected. In the aftermath of her stroke, when Ms. E needs it the most, she is left bereft of the most powerful tool in her meaning-making toolbox, the power of narrative. Yet without this power she is extremely vulnerable to the cascading effects of a catastrophic reaction. Ms. E, we believe, is well acquainted with this vulnerability.

At this point it is timely to recall the three core features that characterize a catastrophic reaction—inconsistent and inadequate behavior, intense anxiety, and dissolution of the self, and evaluate them in terms of the narrative functions we have just covered. We begin with inconsistent and inadequate behavior, or as Goldstein often refered to it, "disordered behavior."

He viewed this type of behavior as being the result of situational demands that are beyond an individual's capabilities. Reformulating this idea from a narrative-psychological perspective, disordered behavior is the result of situational demands that are beyond one's discursive and specifically narrative possibilities. As noted earlier, Ms. E's storytelling is not up to the task of helping her deal with the complex and threatening situation of having a "new" brain. In fact, her narrative reach is limited in more than one respect. This is highly consequential because narrative not only reflects and articulates the newly acquired internal disorder of her damaged cortex, but also contributes to generate it.

The narrative dysfunction that most directly relates to disordered behavior is what we view as the breakdown of coherence in Ms. E's narratives. This implies that she cannot rely on her own interpretations to help her make sense of her situation and act accordingly. Instead, she experiences even more chaos by positing stories that evoke a reality—a reality that is fragmented, directionless, and in a state of constant flux. As mentioned in the previous paragraph, narrative not only speaks *of* experience; it *is* an experience. Another contributor to Ms. E's disordered behavior is that her stories do not allow her to reflect on and evaluate her world in a way that would enable ordered behavior. Insofar as her stories suggest a picture of herself as being the woman she always was, the woman without a stroke, the woman in charge, the strong and healthy woman, they do not work to inform her that her existential being in the world has fundamentally changed. The more she talks, the more this picture comes full circle.

As a result, there is a fundamental incongruence between the narrative reality she lives and the reality of her life as a hospitalized patient. As we saw, she is somehow aware of this incongruence. But none of her stories offers a plausible explanation of the chasm between the different realities in which she lives. Further, none of her narratives creates any distance from the here and now of her everyday life. She finds herself trapped in the immediacy of a stream of consciousness, a stream that envelopes her and makes it impossible to explore any alternative options of thought and behavior. In addition, she cannot rely on other people to support ordered behavior on her behalf because this would depend on an established mode of communication.

How could such a state not lead to extreme anxiety, which Goldstein stressed as the second core feature of a catastrophic reaction? Anxiety does not exist in an affective vacuum but rather is associated with a flood of negative emotions. To be sure, this is the case for Ms. E, who vacillates between anger, sadness, fear, and frustration. As she explains elsewhere in the interview, she feels "lost" and "freaked out." Without being able to support her, we witnessed the devastating impact of this emotional overflow on the structure and content of her stories, and vice versa; how her breathless narrative overflow often pulled her emotional life with it. Although her narratives might have been grossly organized around her emotions, they nevertheless failed to help her deal with her anxiety. Mark Freeman (2008) describes the similarly poignant limits and limitations of narrative in the life of his mother suffering from Alzheimer's disease. For Goldstein, the person does not *have* anxiety but *is* the anxiety. To have anxiety requires distance; the consequence of having no distance is to be anxiety. In the case of Ms. E, because her narratives fall short in distancing her from her immediate experience of herself, she is forced to embody it.

The "dissolution of the self" is the third core feature of a catastrophic reaction. Once again, we can see how narrative both reflects and constitutes experience, in this case, the experience of one's self. The quality of Ms E's mental life has been altered so drastically—even if her narrative's "normalizing" stickiness might aim to convince her otherwise—that she no longer recognizes herself. Indeed, there is a literal truth to her statement "I'm lost." What else can losing oneself in an array of incoherent and fragmented storylines lead to other than to the experience of an incoherent and fragmented self? And finally, how could one expect any help when there is no other in the world, no one to communicate and to connect to?

What can we say, then, about the possible future of Ms. E? Will she ever return from "being lost" and is there a way to recover from a catastrophic reaction? We believe that there might have been a reason for Goldstein not to talk about the "final catastrophe" or a "catastrophic ending" but just about a "catastrophic reaction." Although Ms. E's mental state as manifested at the time of the interview was undoubtedly desperate, this is not necessarily her final state. There may be other, less optimistic views about the future of individuals who went through what we described as catastrophic reaction (see Nochi, 1998). However, roughly a year after Ms. E's catastrophic reaction/narrative breakdown a number of the "symptoms" we examined had subsided. She still talked a lot, but we were sure that her stories had moved her out of the eye of the catastrophe. Whether due to neurological recovery or learning to narrate in new, perhaps more dialogical and communicative ways, it seemed as if her insistence to bring coherence to her shattered world eventually moved her out of the "raging river" and onto firmer ground. "New narrating" has also been observed and can emerge in individuals with memory impairments (see Medved, 2007; Medved & Brockmeier, 2008). It is a strange and puzzling form of discourse that requires more detailed attention, but this is a topic for another chapter.

In conclusion, "symptoms are answers, given by the modified organism, to definite demands: they are attempted solutions" (Goldstein, 1934/1995, p. 35). We propose to understand Ms. E's narratives in a similar way: as attempted solutions, even if such attempts, in the midst of the chaos of a catastrophic reaction, are often frantic and failed attempts at solutions. Nevertheless, such attempts are driven by an obviously unbroken desire to narrate, to search for a way out even in a moment when almost everything seemed dark—a desperate storytelling that tries to cope with the unspeakable and unthinkable.

More than a half-century after Goldstein and in the wake of numerous neuroscientific breakthroughs, Prigatano (1999) observed that the psychological disruption caused by higher cerebral dysfunction is still poorly understood. This has not changed in the new millennium. Given the high proportion of people who are or will suffer impaired neurological functioning in their lifetime, we find this surprising. To alleviate this lack of understanding about the world of individuals with neurotrauma, the study of their broken narratives can shed light on disruptions such as catastrophic reactions, while the study of such disruptions can also shed light on the very workings of narrative meaning-making.

REFERENCES

Brockmeier, J. (2002). Possible lives. *Narrative Inquiry, 12,* 455–466.

Brockmeier, J. (2004). What makes a story coherent? In A. Uchoa Branco & J. Valsiner (Eds.), *Communication and metacommunication in human development* (pp. 285–306). Greenwich, CT: Information Age Publishing.

Brockmeier, J. (2005). Pathways of narrative meaning construction. In B. D. Homer & C. Tamis-LeMonda (Eds.), *The development of social cognition and communication* (pp. 291–313). Mahwah, NJ: Lawrence Erlbaum.

Bruner, J. S. (1990). *Acts of meaning.* Cambridge, MA: Harvard University Press.

Bruner, J. S. (2002). Narrative distancing: A foundation of literacy. In J. Brockmeier, M. Wang, & D. R. Olson (Eds.), *Literacy, narrative and culture* (pp. 86–93). Richmond, UK: Curzon Press.

DeLuca, J., & Diamond, B. J. (1995). Aneursym of the anterior communicating artery: A review of neuroanatomical and neuropsychological sequelae. *Journal of Clinical and Experimental Neuropsychology, 17,* 100–121.

Freeman, M. (2008). Beyond narrative: Dementia's tragic promise. In L. C. Hydén & J. Brockmeier (Eds.), *Illness, health and culture: Broken narratives* (pp. 169–184). New York: Routledge.

Goldstein, K. (1942). *Aftereffects of brain injuries in war.* New York: Grune and Stratton.

Goldstein, K. (1952). The effect of brain damage on the personality. *Psychiatry, 15,* 245–260.

Goldstein, K. (1995). *The organism: A holistic approach to biology derived from pathological data in man.* New York: Zone Books. (Original work published 1934)

Hydén, L.-C. (2008). Vicarious voices. In L. C. Hydén & J. Brockmeier (Eds.), *Illness, health and culture: Broken narratives* (pp. 36–53). New York: Routledge.

Medved, M. I. (2007). Remembering without a past: A study of anterograde memory impairment in individuals after neurotrauma. *Psychology, Health and Medicine, 12,* 603–616.

Medved, M. I., & Brockmeier, J. (2004). Making sense of traumatic experiences: Telling your life with Fragile X syndrome. *Qualitative Health Research, 14,* 741–759.

Medved, M. I., & Brockmeier, J. (2008). Continuity amid chaos: Neurotrauma, loss of memory, and sense of self. *Qualitative Health Research, 18,* 469–479.

Nochi, M. (1998). "Loss of self" in the narratives of people with traumatic brain injuries: A qualitative analysis. *Social Science and Medicine, 46,* 869–878.

Prigatano, G. P. (1999). *Principles of neuropsychological rehabilitation.* New York: Oxford.

Ricoeur, P. (1991). Life in quest of narrative. In D. Wood (Ed.), *On Paul Ricoeur: Narrative and interpretation* (pp. 20–33). London: Routledge.

Sacks, O. (1995). Foreword. In K. Goldstein, *The organism: A holistic approach to biology derived from pathological data in man* (pp. 7–14). New York: Zone Books.

Vygotsky, L. S. (1978). *Mind in society: The development of higher psychological processes.* In M. Cole, V. J. Steiner, S. Scribner, & E. Sauberman (Eds.). Cambridge, MA: Harvard University (Russ. 1930, 1933, & 1935).

Vygotsky, L. S., & Luria, A. (1994). Tool and symbol in child development. In R. van der Veer & J. Valsiner (Eds.), *The Vygotsky reader* (pp. 99–174). Oxford & Cambridge, MA: Blackwell (Russ. 1930).

Young, K., & Saver, J. L. (2001). The neurology of narrative. *Substance: A Review of Theory and Literary Criticism, 30,* 72–84.

5 Stories That are Ready to Break

Cheryl F. Mattingly

When illness is protracted, when there is no chance of return to the person one once was, or when there is no hope of being "normal," a person's very sense of self is lived in a special way through the body. Personal identity becomes intimately tied to the pain, uncertainty, and stigma that come with an afflicted body. What might it mean to be healed when a cure is only a distant possibility or no possibility at all? The inevitable poverty of biomedical responses to this question has a great deal to do with why narrative is so irresistible. Stories, told or acted, offer healing possibilities that reach far beyond the purview of biomedicine. They can help transform identity, interpret the meaning of the past and even provide images of possible futures. This narrative potential has spawned a wealth of scholarship on the relation of narrative, illness, and personal identity. (See, e.g., Bülow & Hydén, 2003; Becker, 1997; Brockmeier, 2002; Cain, 1991; Charon & Montello, 2002; Frank, 1995; Garro, 2000; Good & Good, 1994; Greenhalgh & Hurwitz, 1998; Hydén, 1997; Kleinman, 1988; Medved & Brockmeier, 2004; Monks, 2000; Morris, 1998.) But stories have insidious potential as well, closing down possibilities, cloaking power in the name of "stating the facts," preventing the very changes that might lead to healing. The very form of stories may oppress, forcing a meaning that denies or overrides a chaotic or inarticulate personal experience. Kirmayer, for example, contends that the coherence that is part of a well-told tale can distance the sufferer from her experience of suffering. Stories can be vehicles for ideology making, especially when coconstructed with powerful physicians, producing texts that are, from the patient's point of view, experience distant. Metaphors and "fragmentary stories, narrative strands" may be more revealing than a finely wrought narrative (Kirmayer 2000, p. 171). Unni Wikan (2000) also objects that sometimes stories present life in an overly coherent way and cannot necessarily be called upon when facing an unpredictable illness. It may even be that silences or half-told tales disclose more about what it is like to be flattened by a serious and unexpected illness, to "fall out of one's life," as Gadamer (1996, p. 42) puts it.

The verisimilitude of stories produces another danger. The very seductiveness of stories, the vividness of the concrete detail, can persuade an audience (and the narrator herself) that a story simply recounts what actually happened, just conveys "the facts." Clinicians routinely tell stories, especially upon confronting "difficult cases" where, as they sometimes say, "social factors" are deemed significant, or when a patient has been labeled "non-compliant." In such circumstances, storytelling abounds in clinical work. These narratives are unlikely to be part of the official medical record, but they are a powerful force in guiding the actual practice of clinicians, one rarely subjected to critical reflection. A persuasive story can have greater influence on such key decisions as whether a patient will receive care, be discharged, or referred, than the specifics of the diagnosis (Mattingly, 1998a).

In this chapter, I want to examine narrative neither as something that heals, nor as something that obstructs healing. Rather, I want to look at narrative as a fragile act that, even when it seems most promising as an instrument for healing, can easily be abandoned or undermined in the course of clinical care. I begin this consideration of "fragile narratives" not with stories, but with an experience of trauma and recovery.

When Oliver Sacks fell off a mountain, he found himself in a hospital with a leg that would not move. This temporary paralysis was no mere matter of torn tendons, but an injury to the nerves themselves. "The neural traffic had stopped, so to speak," Sacks tells us, "and the streets of the city were deserted and silent" (1987, p. 65). He appears to his doctors and therapists as a patient with a leg injury, a local affair, but he knows better. He has lost his leg altogether, although, strangely, it is still attached to him. With this loss, his very spirit, his imagining, intending, purposeful self, was endangered. "I had lost the power to 'call' to a part of myself, the power to call *on* a part of myself . . ." (p. 66). It becomes painfully clear to Sacks that what he had initially viewed as a peripheral breakdown was, in fact, a breakdown at the center of things, "not just a lesion in my muscle, but a lesion in me" (p. 67). I will also consider the role of rehabilitation for those who, in one way or another, confront lesions that run all the way to the center of themselves, when bodies become sources of pain or humiliation, or when they have cracked to the core. I investigate a puzzle Sacks raises in trying to understand the perspective of his healers. While he finds that his recovery is full of adventures and dramas, his healers see things as routine. How can this be? he wonders indignantly. How can they speak of his recovery as "uneventful" when "recovery *is* events, a series of wonderful, unpredictable events . . . advents, which are births and re-births" (1987, p. 154, italics in original)?

I take up Sack's puzzle by drawing from my own ethnographic research among a range of clinical professionals, including occupational therapists, physical therapists, physicians, nurses and other pediatric clinicians who treat children with serious illnesses and disabilities. The puzzle Sacks notes becomes ever more complex as one attends to the daily practices, discourses and ideologies of these professionals. My colleagues and I have found the systematic suppression of certain kinds of dramas in clinical settings, especially dramas in which a central character is the patient, who emerges as a complex, socially situated person with her own illness experience and biography. But—and here is the mystery that lies at the core of this paper—I have also found sustained efforts to *cultivate* healing dramas which speak to such a person. Among occupational therapists (those health professionals I know best), there is even a discourse in the form of archetypal "best case" stories which stresses the centrality of such dramas to good practice. Sometimes, in other words, healers in Western biomedical settings *do* seem to recognize that recovery is constituted through "events," and "rebirths"; this recognition translates into conscious efforts to support and foster such recovery dramas. However, support is often short lived, undermined or aborted altogether. Even when such fostering occurs, the treating practitioner who in one moment helps to create a powerful healing drama may in the next moment deny that she has done so, or doubt her own wisdom in pursuing such a path. This paper investigates the rise and fall of healing dramas. When and why are they nurtured by healers? What is it about the nature of rehabilitation practices and clinic culture that makes these dramas so fragile, so easily relinquished or neglected? Why do they crop up in the informal storytelling of some professionals but not in the more "official" discourses, such as the medical chart?

HEALING AS DRAMA

Before considering this mystery, it is worth identifying the qualities associated with the "eventful moment" of recovery. To consider healing dramas in the context of rehabilitation and how they might differ from other "noneventful" moments of recovery, I return briefly to Oliver Sacks and his leg injury, asking how Sacks rediscovers and reclaims a leg which seemed for so long to be not merely injured but vanished altogether. At first he begins to feel "crackles" and "flashes" in his leg, this electrical activity betokening neurological life in this formerly absent region. However, these impulses are not connected to *him*, he tell us, because they are disconnected from all will, intention, or idea. Finally comes the day when Sacks's therapist insists he is to stand. He is to resume his uprightness, to overcome his passive, recumbent posture. But he needs to *imagine* how to move his leg, and this is part of his problem. How is Sacks's imagination to be sparked? What will transform a leg electrified to a leg in action? As it turns out, it is music, which gives life to his leg. One day while trying to walk, he suddenly recalls, or more accurately his body recalls, a piece by Mendelssohn he'd happened to hear the day before, not even a piece he much liked. In this embodied remembering, his leg awakes. "Until the music, there had been no feeling whatever" he writes, "Then, all of a sudden, with no warning whatever . . .came *music*, warm, vivid, alive, moving, personal. . . . And in that moment, when the body became action, the leg, the flesh became quick and alive, the flesh became music, incarnate solid music" (1987, pp. 147–148).

This walk, joyously executed, transforms his first musicless, robotic steps into his own natural rhythm. It marks a turning point in his own recovery. This moment becomes the stuff of which stories can (and will) be told. And what of this momentous walk? Here we have the most ordinary thing taking on dramatic stakes *precisely* at the moment when it resumes its natural place as habitual, unconscious action. His walk shifts from exhausting calculation to thoughtless movement. And what does Sacks recover in this transformative, thoughtless moment? More than a leg. It is himself which is recovered. "It was the triumphant return of the quintessential living 'I'. . ." (p. 149).

This music, recollected by his body kinesthetically through his first faltering steps, engenders an experience that bears the mark of a narrative moment with its own dramatic structure. The experience Sacks describes is something shaped. It presents itself to him as *an* experience, in the language of a certain branch of phenomenology (Gadamer, 1975; Dilthey, 1989). He is not merely living through something, surviving something. He is having *an* experience that can be distinguished from others, that can be partly disclosed in textual form—as, in fact, a story. Every experience has something in it of the idea of adventure, Simmel argued. His experience constitutes a story in the making, an adventure worth telling a story about.

But notice the peculiar ambiguous quality to "experience" here. Whatever Sacks can later say, quite obviously his words can never capture the experience itself as something felt in his body. Even his memories of these dramatic moments are not simple representations of a past. And yet, he has had a singular experience which is indeed preserved in memory and therefore can be returned to, recalled, even reheard, and refelt. Experience, when it emerges as a unique memory-making event, bears an ambiguous quality. It has some of the qualities of an object, inscribed in memory as a particular something which can be represented. And yet it is also fleeting and, as Gadamer says, "inexhaustible" in its potential meaning. It resists representation. Significant experiences can never be captured by any images, any "objects" preserved in text or other medium. The antirepresentational qualities of significant experience also have to do with their practical capabilities; meaning is never fixed because it changes a future, and that future will remake the meaning of the past. Sacks's experience of being "musicked along" by Mendelssohn is not merely remembered, it is remembered as transformative, slicing his life into a "before" and "after." This significant experience, preserved for all his life, becomes generative of new experiences (including the writing of a book about them) which, in turn, imbue new and different meanings on that one moment of recovery. Yet this rebirth via Mendelssohn is also evanescent. It disappears, never to be fully recaptured or relived.

The connection between significant experience and narrative form has been most extensively explored within philosophy, particularly among those influenced by phenomenological and hermeneutic traditions. Some have suggested that experience itself, or at least significant experience, has narrative form (Carr, 1986, 1997; Crites, 1997; Ricoeur, 1983, 1984; Olafson, 1979; MacIntyre, 1981). Related arguments concerning the human propensity to understand and interpret ongoing actions by seeing them as parts of unfolding narratives have arisen in various branches of cognitive, psychoanalytic, and developmental psychology (cf. Bruner, 1986, 1990, 1991; Polkinghorne, 1988; Stern, 1994, 1995).

Within anthropology, the link between drama, narrative and healing has been explored by those who analyze non-Western and alternative healing rituals. However, there has been little attention to the formal qualities of *narrative* and those significant experiences that are often at the heart of the healing ritual. Anthropological studies of healing rituals underscore that most significant experiences do not simply befall humans but are carefully crafted and staged, sometimes even rehearsed. They are, in short, created as well as received. Both creation and reception are a social affair. Healing rituals across a wide array of cultures have been noted for features, which, I will try to show, are also integral to the power and efficacy of these "hidden dramas" within biomedical practice:

1. There is a heightened attention to the moment, an "existential immediacy" which gives an authority and legitimacy to the activity (Csordas, 1996, 1994; Schieffelin, 1996; Desjarlais, 1996).
2. A multiplicity of communicative channels carry the meaning, creating a "fusion of experience" (Briggs, 1996; Tambiah, 1985).
3. Aesthetic, sensuous, and extra-linguistic qualities of the interaction are accentuated (Stoller, 1989, 1996, 1997; Laderman, 1996; Jackson, 1989).
4. The intensification of experience is socially shared, and it emerges through mutual bodily engagement with others (Kapferer, 1983, 1986; Danforth, 1989; Schechner, 1990; Hughes-Freeland, 1998).
5. Healing actions are symbolically dense, creating images which refer both backward and forward in time—the patient is located symbolically in history (Kendall, 1996).
6. Efficacy is linked to potential transformations of the "patient" and sometimes a larger social community (Kendall, 1996; Turner, 1969, 1986a, 1986b; Turner, 1992).

For a more extended discussion of these qualities as aspects of Western biomedical practice, see Mattingly (2000).

The ephemeral character of significant and memory-making experience which has intrigued philosophers takes on added complexities when examined from an anthropological standpoint in which the role of culture and social context is factored in. The fleeting quality of Sacks's recovery experience is no mere existential given. It is abetted because Sacks's experience is largely private, interior, despite strenuous efforts to involve those around him. His doctors, nurses and therapists are unaware (or find insignificant) what has happened to him. Sacks has his narrative moments, his astonishing experiences, but he apparently has them all by himself. He experiences dramas, stories in the making, where the professionals see only a mundane, predictable path. When he steals a look at his chart and finds written "uneventful recovery," he concludes that his healers are "mad." In turning to our own research, we explore the aesthetic, embodied, highly charged and narratively shaped qualities of recovery events and their centrality to healing. The "madness" shows up as well, a point I also explore in the context of my own research in pediatric rehabilitation practice.

HIDDEN DRAMAS IN PEDIATRIC PRACTICE

My data are drawn from two ethnographic studies of pediatric health care, one in Chicago and the second in Los Angeles. The Chicago study, conducted between 1994 and 1996, involved 10 pediatric occupational therapists, their young patients and, where possible, parents and other key family members. Mary Lawlor and I, along with a team of other research colleagues, carried out the study in two clinical sites located in the heart of the city, one in the downtown area, the other on the near west side. These two hospitals serve populations overwhelmingly African-American and Mexican-American and low income. We observed and, when possible, videotaped clinical encounters. We have also interviewed therapists and family members, audiotaping and subsequently transcribing these interviews. The focus of the study was to examine "therapeutic partnering" with patients and families. Rehabilitation, particularly in out-patient pediatrics, requires high levels of collaboration and support among therapists, patients, and key family care givers who are asked to carry out "home programs" involving exercises and other therapeutic treatments. In this study we were primarily focused on the therapist's perceptions of what constituted effective collaboration with children and families, how they went about trying to create it, and their perception of dilemmas and obstacles to their effectiveness. Where we were able to obtain permission from families, we separately interviewed parents (or primary family care giver) and the children participating in the study.

The second study, located primarily in two clinical sites in Los Angeles, also addresses the issue of collaboration among health care providers, patients and family members, but on a much larger scale. Here again, Mary Lawlor and I have served as primary collaborators, but have developed a team of researchers who have been instrumental. This 9-year study, begun in 1997 and still ongoing, is built upon the design and some findings that grew out of the Chicago research. It, too, examines communication and collaboration among children, healthcare practitioners and families. However, it is a much broader study in several senses. It focuses equally on healthcare professionals and the institutional cultures in which care takes place and on the children and families who receive services. Though we entered both clinical sites through contacts with occupational therapists, and these professionals have been more extensively followed than other health care practitioners, the study includes a very broad array of health professionals: surgeons, oncologists, radiologists, pediatricians, social workers, nurses, nutritionists, physical therapists, speech therapists, health care aides, special educational teachers, psychologists. It also goes well beyond the Chicago research by following children and families outside the clinical encounter into their homes, schools, and neighborhoods. In fact, while there is still extensive time spent at the two clinic sites where the families were initially recruited, the central actors in the study are the 30 African-American children and their families. Once families agreed to participate, healthcare professionals were recruited on the basis of their involvement with the children and families. Since the total sample is quite large (well over 500) and data collection tends to be intensive (with multiple interviews, observations, and videotapes), we have not been conducting this research alone. We have assembled a core research team, including doctoral students and recent doctoral graduates in both anthropology and occupational science and therapy.

The 9-year longitudinal ethnography has allowed us to follow children and families as they change. This, too, while making for a more complicated study, has offered a much deeper understanding of what turns out to make a difference in the partnering efforts of healthcare professionals and families. It has enabled us to connect minute intense moments of "significant experience" and minor healing dramas which never show up in the medical chart to the lives of children and families beyond the clinical encounter.

The children in the Los Angeles study, like those in the Chicago study, do not share a single kind of disease or disability. Rather, they share certain commonalities of "illness experience," suffering from a serious, chronic illness, or disability that requires frequent visits to an array of healthcare professionals and substantial efforts by family members to provide care at home. In addition, since this study focuses exclusively on African-Americans children, there is a shared ethnic/racial label. As might be expected, there is substantial diversity as well in the families that comprise our sample group. However, certain patterns appear across the cases. The importance of powerful healing dramas in the rehabilitation process, and their significance to children and families, for example, is broadly shared. Since the vast majority of health care providers in our sites are not themselves African-American and are from middle and upper income strata, collaboration between professionals and families means connecting across cultural worlds and racial boundaries where wariness and suspicion often create a subtle undercurrent of tension.

The two cases I analyze (one from each study) were selected because they illustrate the dramatic and aesthetic qualities of quite ordinary treatment interventions in rehabilitation. Also, they reveal the paradox which is central to this paper and figures prominently in our data: the way that healing dramas are at once cultivated and suppressed by pediatric health professionals. This paradox shows up in numerous forms. Treatment goals emphasize "fixing" or improving body parts but when practitioners describe what they think really matters about their interventions, they are likely to stress the importance of using therapy time to encourage dramatic transformations in the perspectives and practices of patients and family members. Occupational and physical therapists who are particularly adept at encouraging children to engage in highly creative activities, embedding exercises designed to "treat an arm" or "improve gross motor coordination" within imaginative scenarios that delight the children they treat, will speak dismissively of these efforts in subsequent interviews. "You know, with kids, you really have to motivate them or they won't work in therapy," they explain with some embarrassment when they have resorted to creative and playful treatment programs. Higher status practitioners who themselves find creative ways to connect with children and families will critique colleagues and subordinates for spending too much time "just playing" with children instead of "getting the work done." Talking and playing are typically set against exercises, procedures and other "real work" features of clinical practice such that the former are perceived to take time away from the latter. Clinicians facilitating powerful healing dramas readily discharge the children rather than make the case to colleagues or families for continued treatment. Short stays and early discharges are, of course, readily traced to a reimbursement system largely out of the hands of individual clinicians. The irony here is not that children are discharged too soon but that clinicians (at least occupational therapists and physical therapists) consistently abandon their own powerful work. That is, their own representations of their practice, even in interviews, are characteristically deeply ambivalent. Furthermore, their clinical actions and decisions are often marked by this same ambivalence.

The paradoxical movement to both cultivate and abandon healing dramas is explored in concrete ethnographic detail below. The clinicians who are the main protagonists in these dramas are occupational therapists. The children are from low-income, urban communities typical of the population served by the clinical sites (Latino and African-American). The children in the two cases both suffer not only from a disabling physical condition but arrive for treatment laden with a welter of behavioral, cognitive, and emotional disorders and these play a major role in the unfolding dramas.

Felicia and the Raven-Haired Pocohontas

One winter day at a hospital in Chicago, Mary Lawlor and I observed a session in which an occupational therapist, Penny, was treating a young teenaged girl of about 13 or 14. We will call her Felicia. Felicia had been referred by special educators at her school for treatment at this out-patient clinic. Once a week Felicia was bused from school to the hospital for therapy. The therapist told us in a later interview something of the diagnostic history that brought her to occupational therapy which included leukemia when she was 8 or 9, which was in remission, seizure disorders, and a fuzzy psychiatric diagnosis, which the therapist variously called "oppositional defiant disorder" and "conduct disorder." The particular problems Penny, the therapist, was to address were some delays in fine motor and visual motor skills. Felicia's teachers especially wanted the therapist to work on her handwriting, which was very messy.

At the time of the session, the therapist had known Felicia for about 2 years. They had a very close relationship. Felicia was the only one in her school who got to go to occupational therapy and this made her feel special. She also enjoyed what they did in occupational therapy, which was mostly a lot of craft projects and some handwriting and computer writing work. While Felicia missed a lot of school, she never missed Fridays. The therapist said that she would "always beg her father on Thursday night to make sure that he woke her up for Friday because she didn't want to miss O.T."

Here is the scene we observed when we first met Felicia. In she walks to the occupational therapy treatment room, a bouncy and rather large girl, a little unkempt but with a tremendously friendly smile. There is an initial struggle between Penny and Felicia about which activity they will do in therapy. Penny has offered Felicia the option of one among several possible prepackaged sand painting kits. The outside boxes show pictures of the finished paintings (all Disney characters from various movies) and Felicia pores carefully over each one. This initial scene between Penny and Felicia is keyed playfully but with a serious undertone, in which the therapist is trying to speed Felicia along, clearly with an eye to their limited time. Felicia makes a great show of indecisiveness, and even seems to be teasing Penny. "Jeez, don't rush me!" she says with a great laugh and a conspiratorial grin to the two unknown observers huddled in the corner watching the scene with their notebooks open. Finally things settle down, and we see that, at the therapist's urging, they are going to do a sand painting of Pocahontas. This Pocahontas, in the finished illustration featured on the cover, is a very pretty slim girl of about 16 with many brightly colored birds circling her head like a kind of halo. All about her is a very blue sky. Penny and Felicia settle at a small table with their kit and now prepare to get started. They immediately contest just how they are going to organize the task. Shall they line up the colored packets of sand by their numbers (Penny's preference)? Or by those which just seem to fit together (Felicia's scheme)?

Finally, 10 or 15 minutes into the session, things get going. Felicia gradually becomes absorbed, pouring the sand with painstaking care, surveying her work with a critical eye. She appears to have forgotten her audience entirely. She is silent, intent, crafting her picture, with occasional guidance from the therapist. A few minutes later, they color Pocahontas's hair, which makes up a large patch of the picture. This is glossy, shiny black hair. Silky and long. The therapist says to Felicia, "She's very pretty." They both agree. "She has hair like yours!" Penny then tells her. I note later to Mary that she was completely startled at this. The therapist is right. Felicia may not be the beautiful Pocahontas but she has exactly her hair. The same silky blue-black hair of this fairy tale girl surrounded by these lovely birds. When Mary and I reconnoiter later in the hospital cafeteria, they return to this moment in this session. I say, "So, they weren't really painting Pocahontas; they were creating a mirror, a fairy tale mirror, of who Felicia might be. The beautiful girl she is not but might imagine herself to be. They are making a mirror, an image of one possible future image." We suddenly recognize that Felicia could be quite pretty. We resee her in our minds. We begin to see this session as a place where pictures are made. These are not most importantly literal ones, but rather imaginative ones where images are created and negotiated.

The activities of Penny and Felicia create a sort of image, a kinesthetic image of concentration and focus required to craft something Felicia finds worth creating. Felicia shifts from being a bouncy but tendentious girl to one who concentrates carefully, head bent, completely focused on her task. A girl who has the skills and desire to create something that brings her pleasure—someone who can sit still long enough to do a good job. And the picture itself, however foolish and fantastical, offers another image. It is not just any picture, but a picture of a girl not so much older than Felicia herself, and with that same abundance of rich black hair. Felicia, when she smiles, even gives off something of Pocahontas's cheery brilliance. (In fact, there is something preferable about the impishness of Felicia's grin when compared to the blank beauty of the Walt Disney character.) But look at Pocahontas! Loved by all, even the birds. Free to wander under a clear sky. Not trapped in a dark, cold apartment in a Chicago winter babysitting three young children and fattening up on potato chips, the image Penny sees when she looks fearfully into Felicia's future. Pocahontas may have her troubles but her world certainly sparkles. Penny doesn't mean to pass along fairytales to Felicia. In fact, it bothers her that Felicia, at her age, is still so enamored of these magical figures. She notes in a later interview that Felicia "always like tends to pick things that are pretty like that . . . more immature for her age . . . and fairy tale scenes. . . ." And Penny worries a little that she allows Felicia to select therapeutic activities which are "7-, 8-, 9-year-old type things . . . if you compare her to other girls 14 and 15, you know, they'd be more into music or whatever."

Yet she helps Felicia to create magical and pretty worlds, magical girls like Pocahontas in these moments of therapy time which have come to mean so much to Felicia. Though Penny doesn't quite seem to realize it, what gets created here is not so much a picture but an *event,* an event that signals possibility. Here is a little drama with qualities associated with healing rituals: a multimedia, symbolically freighted, dramatic, compelling, social creation. The resonance between this present moment and Felicia's past and future emerges even more clearly after interviews with the therapist.

This session is a short story in a larger life story still very much unfolding and where the ending is not at all certain. For compare Pocahontas to the fate Penny fears for Felicia. Penny states that Felicia has "self-esteem problems," speaks of herself as looking "yucky." And Penny tells a terrifying story of a meeting between school professionals, hospital therapists, and parents when she meets Felicia's mother for the first time. She describes her as a tall stern woman who "yells" at all the school and therapy professionals, tells them they don't understand her daughter, and announces she is keeping Felicia for home schooling rather than sending her to school. Felicia hangs her head during this meeting, sitting in a corner. When Penny must leave early, Felicia begs to go with her so that Penny takes her out of the meeting. The therapist also recounts her final session with Felicia (the week after the one we observed) when they just go sit and talk. Felicia, for the first time, talks about her home life in real detail. She, her mother and father, her 2-year-old niece and two brothers all live in a one-bedroom apartment. The therapist, hand held over her heart, offers her picture of Felicia in a few years. Felicia already is primarily responsible for caring for her niece, a 2-year-old left by Felicia's older sister who is never home. The therapist imagines her, the designated family babysitter, eating potato chips and sitting in front of the TV, year in and year out. This is her dark, fearful vision.

Penny is simultaneously helping Felicia address a series of discrete difficulties she faces (for example, paying attention, doing a job well, remembering things, coordinating her physical movements) with a larger project. Penny labels it "building her self-esteem." Certainly that is part of it. But perhaps we could also say that Penny believes Felicia may lack a picture of her future self which is hopeful, which would help guide her in finding the best possible life for herself. Put differently, we might say that Felicia lacks a picture of herself which helps her to see her own possibilities and strengths. Pocahontas may not be a very realistic alternative, but the ability to create Pocahontas, to make, with your hands, a beautiful magical mirror, such an experience may beget other sorts of creations. One need not accept Penny's version of Felicia's life but there are many indicators, just in the single session offered here that this is "an experience" for Felicia. It is not a singular momentous event, like the one described by Sacks, but in its quiet way, it presents a striking image which Felicia just may take home.

On the one hand, Penny is confident that she offers something important and unique to Felicia. She tells us she was "that one special person to do something with." Penny, in her early 20s at the time and with a girlish air, believes Felicia saw her as a kind of "friendly older sister." Felicia has also treated her as a protector on occasion; during the one time Penny met Felicia's mother at a team meeting, a woman whose anger frankly frightened Penny, Felicia shrank away, grabbing Penny's hand for comfort. Where is the fragility in this healing drama? Penny lacks conviction that her work has anything to do with healing. She agrees with team members that Felicia should be discharged from therapy. In the end, Penny does not know how to defend her work with Felicia. Perhaps it really was, as she put it "just a social thing." After all, she readily admits, Felicia's handwriting had never improved in 2 years, and that was a main treatment goal of their work. She speaks sadly of the plans she and Felicia had made about future therapy together. "We also did a lot of work on the computer because her handwriting was so sloppy and there really wasn't, that was not going to change. That had been worked on for 3 years and in school everyday. So we started working on the computer and doing typing and hoping that maybe this could be a way that in the future she could be working and, you know, doing a vocational program or something. So, we had talked about doing, making a newspaper which I had started with another one of the day school kids that she knew about."

Not only is Felicia discharged from therapy, Felicia's mother has decided to take her out of the school program. She tells the professional team she wants to give Felicia home schooling instead, a decision which deeply disturbed Penny. In our final interview with Penny, as she spoke of Felicia's future, tears came to her eyes. She was clearly haunted by this case. A year later, Penny decided to leave pediatric practice because she found it just too emotionally difficult.

Penny might have strongly advocated that Felicia stay in therapy, particularly since she was going to be home schooled and would lose most other contact with the world outside her family. Perhaps Penny might not have won this battle, but she doesn't even try. Furthermore, despite her terrible visions for Felicia's future, she seems to find the recommendations of colleagues for Felicia's discharge reasonable. Why? I could go a certain way in answering this by pointing toward a culture of biomedicine in which illness is defined in narrow diagnostic terms and rehabilitation is identified with well specified procedures that can be judged against clearly observable, ideally measurable, gains in function. But there are more factors at play in the clinical world which support the abandonment of healing dramas, as will be seen shortly.

The Witch's Tea Party

For nearly a year, Vanessa took Leia to emergency rooms all over the city, seeking some kind of diagnosis for her increasingly ill child. Time and time again, she was told to go home, that nothing was really wrong. Finally, after Vanessa's very strong protests that she would not go home until someone looked at her daughter because she knew something was very wrong, a doctor examined her and recognized that there was a serious problem.

Within two days, Leia was diagnosed with a brain tumor that had grown unchecked for a year and was, by the time of diagnosis, the "size of an egg." Prognosis was not good; no more than 60% chance of recovery, the doctors told Vanessa. Leia had surgery and radiation, followed by chemotherapy.

After surgery, Vanessa and her Leia spend at 2 days a week at the hospital for the next year and a half. Tuesdays are chemo. Thursdays are out-patient physical and occupational therapy. Her oncologist is someone Vanessa gradually comes to trust, and there is a physical therapist who Leia is particularly fond of. Vanessa credits this physical therapist with teaching Leia to walk again after surgery, a healing drama of momentous proportions when one hopes for a child to recover. And Leia loves her therapy days because (a) she does not get a shot; and (b) she gets a chance to play with some new people who, sometimes at least, know how to have fun. I describe a moment when a narrative is created in a treatment session with one of her occupational therapists—a narrative which is both hopeful, and, in a sense "ready to break."

An occupational therapist, Amy, who was not so familiar with Leia had just taken over the case. She tried for a few sessions, very unsuccessfully, to get Leia involved in some fine motor activities, like cutting and pasting pictures from magazines onto a page in some collage art activity. Leia was generally bored and fretful, repeatedly jumping up from the table to wander off and see what other toys might be around. About the third frustrating session, Amy had an idea. She noticed that Leia gravitated to some of the play clothes kept in the cupboards of the little treatment room where they had had their sessions. Also, Leia was obsessed with the sink in the treatment room, each session heading immediately to it to wash her hands and then proceeding to take the sponge and wipe down the counters. Amy decided they should have a tea party, in fact a witch's tea party. Leia was delighted. They tried on many clothes together, Leia attempting to tie various scarves on her bald head, preening in front of the mirror, and then settling with great delight on wearing a gigantic black witch's hat. The therapist, Amy, similarly donned a hat and Leia even found one for me to wear, though I was trying to sit quietly in the corner and take notes. They set the table, placing their dishes just so, invited a few stuffed bears and other creatures to the tea, filled the teapot with water (Leia's favorite part) and had some lovely plastic bagels to go with their drinks, which they sipped decorously in a ladylike way. There were, of course, many fine motor components to the party, (scarve tying, buttons buttoned) which was a great hit.

HOW TO THROW A WITCH'S TEA PARTY: THE NARRATIVE EMPLOTMENT OF A THERAPY SESSION

The interlude just recounted marks a shift from a therapy time the therapist designates as "scattered" to a focused and dramatic moment, narrative time governed by a desire, suspense, drama, and a sense of the whole. Play clothes and plastic bagels transform the pair into festive witches eating and drinking with friends. Few words are spoken but this is a story all the same, and one imbued with symbolic density, a story that signifies. The depth of its signifying power is never guessed at by the therapist who so beautifully orchestrates it. Understanding why this therapeutic moment holds power for Leia and her mother depends upon knowing more about Leia's life than this therapist does. However, the therapist is fully aware that she and Leia have effected a transformation in this part of the session. They have managed to shift from clinical time which is scattered, where she cannot get minimal cooperation from Leia, and where, if she is unlucky and this persists, she may have to force Leia to perform a set of tasks directed to discrete problems (weakness of her left side and especially her left hand, attention deficits caused either by the original tumor or brain damage from the surgery). She knows that out of an inauspicious beginning, they move into imaginative play where treatment of pathology is embedded within such merry adventures as dressing up as witches and pouring water from a teapot.

The drama relies upon their ability to move into a cultural script they share, one surrounding the everyday business of making tea and throwing parties. They make tea, they prepare snacks, they share food and drink with others. For this purpose, water becomes tea, stuffed creatures become honored party guests, and plastic bagels the tasty snacks fit for a proper witch's tea. The therapist's ability to follow the "pacing" of Leia and to build opportunistically on what intrigues her, allow all of us—as actors or audience—to enter the "same story"—to create a healing story—for the space of a therapy session. But it is only when placed in context of Leia's (and Vanessa's) unfolding life that the real drama is revealed. This session connects Leia to everyday life in the sense that it plays out a familiar canonical scene. (Leia, like other children her age, loves nothing more than playing at being grown up and cooking is a quintessential everyday activity reserved for those older than herself.) But its dramatic potency is due to the way it disconnects; it creates a breach from the life Leia has been living since her illness. Amy and Leia make an upside down story of her life—one which connects to Leia's life but is powerful for Leia because there are so many reversals of everyday life.

This little performed narrative connects clinic life to a hopeful plot Vanessa is fiercely trying to live out, despite the devastating losses that have recently occurred. This story is one where Leia has a joyful childhood, where she lives to the fullest. This hopeful plot requires such nurturing because it runs counter to the life story that has been unfolding. It is an upside down story in light of the many losses of her recent life. Here is a brief catalogue of the most important ones: (a) she leaves preschool, which she loves, and stays home all the time, away from her friends; (b) her father moves out and her parents are now divorcing; (c) she and her mother move from a small rental house to an apartment because her mother has been fired (missing too many days due to Leia's illness) and can no longer pay the rent on the house; (d) since they are now cramped for space, her 23-year-old sister, who had been living at home, moves out, taking her son who is Leia's age and is very close to Leia; (e) Leia loses her old neighborhood and now lives in a place with no yard; (f) Leia's grandmother is diagnosed with stomach cancer and has become quite ill. She cannot visit Leia as much as she once did; (g) Leia eats so little, has grown so thin from the illness and the chemotherapy, that her mother now gives her a baby bottle because she will eat more that way. Leia seems to be hurtling backward in developmental time.

Leia cries sometimes at the loss of school playmates, father, and nephew, and is frequently mutinous at her mother's constant entreaties that she eat. Eating has become something of a battle between the two of them, and food has become a source of worry rather than fun. And in the midst of what has felt like a losing battle to get Leia to eat, to keep enough food in her, and keep her from losing more weight, this therapy session has offered her a chance to feed others. As a witch at a tea party, she is the nurturer of other creatures as well as herself. She prepares the food and sets the table and brings everyone together. And she does so in disguise. She is Leia but not Leia, for she has donned a mask, a new costume, a new identity—Leia the friendly witch. And she is not at a tea party by herself—what kind of party would that be—but with another witch, the friendly therapist who has finally thought up something fun to do. Even the outside anthropologist is invited to join, as Leia insists that she wear a witch's hat too. So Leia, who loves people but has been spending more and more time alone, can also orchestrate this social gathering, this social drama—thanks to the clever organization by Amy, the therapist.

As Penny does with Felicia, Amy embeds certain activities directed to discrete disabilities (lack of fine motor coordination for Felicia, an impaired left side for Leia) within an activity which she knows the child finds absorbing. And in both cases, the most intense moments are dramatic in their quietude. Time slows. Within this pause, it is possible to glimpse a different child. This glimpse is intensely in the present, which takes on its own authority. But the very intensity of the present facilitates a foreshadowing gaze. This is not a predictive gaze so much as a freewheeling speculation; Felicia enters the body of an Indian princess and Leia is transformed into a cheerful witch capable of caretaking. These are not realistic images. But as with many non-Western healing rituals, their very fancifulness lends them power and intensity—even a certain seductive authority. Perhaps Felicia *will* find her way out of a dark apartment and a life of babysitting. Perhaps Leia *will* emerge from a scary, isolated world where she is not only weighted down with a life threatening illness, but faces the losses of friends and loved ones as well.

FRAIL DRAMAS: THE INVISIBILITY OF HEALING MOMENTS

We do not know what has happened to Felicia but we do know something about the impact of these small dramas on the ability of Leia and Vanessa to create hope. Although the therapists may not realize, their work has helped Vanessa to envision a "return to life" after surgery, in which Leia is able to laugh, walk, and play. In fact, Vanessa sees these therapeutic interventions as so pivotal to Leia's well-being that, unbeknownst to the therapists, she has built an entire home version of the rehab gym.

In this example, the therapist is well attuned to Leia, but she is not at all aware of how her work fits into the larger life world of this child. She, and the other therapists who work with Leia, are fully unaware of the extent to which Leia's mother has incorporated the work of the therapists into her home life. The four therapists I interviewed about Vanessa strongly concurred (in separate interviews) on several points: (a) Vanessa "loved her child to death"; (b) She "popped in and out of sessions," which several therapists found troublesome since all struggled hard to hold Leia's attention and Leia frequently looked for her mother. Often she didn't come to the session at all but disappeared, which also disconcerted or annoyed the therapists; (c) Vanessa seemed "pretty overwhelmed," a phrase repeated by all the therapists. As one put it, "I just think there's lot more going on in her life. She's just got such a full plate. I just get the impression that she's really overwhelmed."; (d) Noting Vanessa's devastation at her child's illness and her life, which has become overwhelming, these therapists often mentioned that Vanessa did not appear to be "absorbing" much of what the therapists were telling her. She often seemed rather "dazed" or "spacey" they said.

These remarks were made in sympathetic tones, a sympathy quite lacking when therapists describe parents *not* perceived as "loving their children to death." However, Vanessa commits a breach from what, in the context of clinic culture, is approved parent behavior. She neither sits through the entire session, nor waits patiently in the waiting room to be called upon by therapists as needed. Instead, she "pops in and out" and "disappears" for stretches at a time. Therapists have few means for evaluating whether parents are good "partners" or not; being available for therapists is an important (and generally unspoken) rule. The "good parent" shows up on time and cooperates with the therapist, assisting, watching from the sidelines, or waiting in another room, as the therapist deems most appropriate. Vanessa's violation of this cultural code requires a narrative explanation. The therapists' story about her life that explains this violation (she "needs a break," she is "overwhelmed," she "has a full plate") is quite correct, as far as it goes. They have read with unerring acuity Vanessa's love for her child and guessed with equal accuracy that there are many more difficulties Vanessa faces.

What they have missed, in their sympathetic reading, is Vanessa's capacity to be overwhelmed, to violate the cultural code of the out-patient rehabilitation unit, and still be able to "read" their minds, to see what they are doing and why it is important for her child. They are utterly unaware of the extent to which Vanessa has gone beyond anything they would dream of asking in incorporating therapy life into home life. Vanessa views all the rehabilitation therapies as utterly central to her quest to, in effect, bring Leia back to life after her surgery. When I have asked Vanessa what she thinks the point of therapy is, she always returns to a moment after Leia's initial surgery, painting a vivid picture of how therapy, as well as her family, has helped to bring Leia back to life. Therapy's role is to get Leia "back to where she was before she got bad. Because," she explains, "after the surgery was over, she could not even walk. She could not use her hands, well at least her left hand. She could not use her left eye. So she couldn't do anything . . . when she, you know, was out of surgery and they moved her downstairs, it was like she couldn't do nothing but just lay there. She wouldn't even laugh until my grandson and my father came up here to the hospital. And then, she like, my grandson was making her laugh and she was like starting laughing. She got all in good spirits. . . . She just started laughing and she was coming, like coming back to life."

In Vanessa's narrative of Leia's "return to life" after surgery, the therapists are instrumental, even helping her to walk again, one of those recovery moments that are always dramatic for parents. At one point, in remarkable synchrony with many of the therapists' accounts of how they work with children, Vanessa relies on musical metaphor to depict the skill of the therapists. Jane (Leia's favorite physical therapist) was so good with Leia because she tried to "fall into Leia's mode of behavior." The therapists were good because they knew how to "slow down" and "take time" with Leia. They push Leia because they are able to figure her out. In a truly Brunerian depiction, Vanessa describes herself watching Jane watching Leia and she says, laughingly of Jane, that she could "read her mind."

What would most astonish the therapists is not only Vanessa's accuracy at reading what they have been doing, and why it matters, but how thoroughly she has built upon their work. She is, in fact, the dream parent, the one that therapists long for. She has transformed her entire living room in her small one-bedroom apartment. It looks like a compressed version of the large rehabilitation room in the outpatient clinic. There is a child-sized basketball hoop, a slide, tunnels to crawl through, even a cheaper version of a "ball bath," a standard piece of pediatric rehabilitation equipment. Vanessa remarked, who saw nothing extraordinary in what she'd done, explained matter of factly that she thought it would be good for Leia to have this set-up at home so that Leia could work more on the therapeutic activities Vanessa had seen the therapists do with her at the hospital. She laughingly noted that Leia's cousins and nephew were her "home therapists" because they got her to play on all the equipment.

It is not just Vanessa who tries to create experiences in which the hopeful stories born in therapy are lived out. Leia, too, looks for such opportunities. And when the occupational therapist has the good sense to offer the chance for a witch's tea party, Leia takes full advantage, laughing as she admires herself in her extravagant witch's hat. This is a particular way to consider "learning by doing" or "learning from experience," where the task to be learned is an emotion, if you want to put it that way, a whole perspective on life.

Life is complex and it would be foolish to presume these few months of occupational therapy sessions with Amy as single-handedly altering Leia's fortunes. But at the very least, it is clear that Amy helps Leia and her mother to realize an image that is mostly hidden by her poor physical health, her grim prognosis, and her difficult home situation.

One plausible story to tell about Leia and Amy is that Amy played a vital role in cultivating hopeful possibilities for Leia and her family. She saw something in this child at a time when the predictions of other health-care professionals were grim. Better and more important, she could use what she saw or guessed about Leia to help create dramas in which this picture was embodied, was made evident to everyone: mother, researcher, Leia herself.

And yet, for all of the brilliance of Amy's work with this child, there is a fragility that surrounds her interventions. While she recognizes her success in building fine motor skills, she fails to recognize the significance of these interventions in recrafting a tragic vision of Leia's future into the hopeful possibility of a "return to life." These failures are very like Penny's, failures of omission one might say, in which the charmed and potent experiences created in therapy are not seen, or are readily relinquished. One moral here, for health professionals, is that even when it is not clear what significance a session has, even when the parent doesn't seem to be around, it is possible, very possible, that more is going on than even meets the clinician's eye. It is possible that clinicians, more often and more powerfully than they even realize, may be contributing to the creation of life stories, offering hopeful moments with deep phenomenological impart. What is it about the clinic culture which propels these two different therapists, working in two different cities, to cultivate and then abandon the healing dramas they set in motion?

THE SUPPRESSION OF HEALING DRAMAS
IN PEDIATRIC PRACTICE

The healing dramas we have described very often pass unnoticed or are abandoned by their creators for a number of reasons directly connected to the culture of the clinical world. Most obvious is the organizing role of the diagnosis in framing what constitutes appropriate treatment. The cases of Leia and Felicia (with their multiple disabilities) reveal a *hierarchy* among diagnostic categories, with some diagnoses more "real" and more deserving of clinical attention than others. The power of any particular diagnosis is not necessarily linked to its impact on a patient's overall health, but rather on its symbolic (and economic) capital. This, in turn, is closely linked to another kind of hierarchy—the power and ranking of the diagnostician who has "awarded" the diagnosis to a particular patient. Felicia's situation illustrates. Here is a girl whose behavioral problems and lack of self-esteem have a far greater negative impact on her life than her occasional seizures and dormant leukemia. However, the behavioral and emotional disabilities have been diagnosed by school psychologists and occupational therapists while her medical diagnoses are the province of medical professionals with much higher status.

Technology and specialized training play a key part in determining the symbolic capital of any given diagnosis. Anthropologists have repeatedly underscored the technology-driven nature of Western biomedicine and the insidious ill effects of health care which is built around such technology (Davis-Floyd & Davis, 1996; Jordan, 1993). Psychologists and therapists practice comparatively "low tech" medicine but surgeries, like the removal of Leia's brain tumor are extremely intricate. Many medical practitioners admit that rehabilitation (those low technology interventions offered by therapists) is critical to the functional outcome of the medical procedures they perform. Nonetheless, many of these same practitioners will argue that it is the more traditional biomedical interventions, such as surgeries, which lend a particular diagnosis its status and justifies hospital treatment. The institutional hierarchy may set rehabilitation therapists such as Penny and Amy against much more powerful professionals, lending to a hesitancy to pursue concerns over comparatively low status diagnostic problems.

Notably, the kind of rehabilitation program many biomedical professionals have in mind does not involve the playful, imaginative, and dramatic moments which therapists like Amy excel at creating. In fact, some doctors depict themselves as continually waging a battle with the rehabilitation therapists to put in more of their time doing "stretching" and other exercises directed at the injured site rather than spending their time *"merely playing"* with children. What I had seen as effective drama, the creation of a healing experience that did much more than allow Felicia to concentrate on a task, Penny feared that this would be seen by other professionals as "just a social thing." The difficulty is not simply that from the institutional perspective, Penny should not be focusing on Felicia's self-esteem. There is a concern among physicians that rehabilitation therapists focus on goals directly tied to surgeries and other medical procedures. Doctors are, in this sense, dependent upon the actions of the lower status professionals and patients themselves, for their interventions to be successful.

The link between healing and technology in Western biomedical practices becomes evident in a different sense when one looks at those health care practices where the "hands on" skill of the professional is the primary tool for treatment. Biomechanical metaphors apply not merely to the body of the patient, but also to the healer as well. Rehabilitation therapists are often viewed, and view themselves, as technicians of the body, as easily interchangeable providers of technical interventions. Key decisions about intervention are often made apart from what the actual healer might determine as necessary. Furthermore, therapists like Penny doubt that the non-"technical" aspects of their work are justifiable forms of treatment.

There is also the valorization of the routine as against the dramatic within clinic culture. Cutting-edge surgeries may attract media coverage, but as anthropologists have pointed out, modern clinics are organized in a way to make even the newest and most experimental interventions *appear* routine. Biomedical practices are carried out in an institutional atmosphere of routineness. Medical professionals find ways to routinize their practice and thus, metaphorically at least, bring the unruly and frightening world of illness under control. Illness is, by nature, an unpredictable thing and much of medicine is fraught with uncertainty (Becker, 1994; Hunter, 1991). The need to control illness is an endemic issue (Becker & Kaufman, 1995; Rhodes, 1993). In biomedical practices, argue Davis-Floyd & Davis, "A reassuring cultural order is imposed on the otherwise frightening and potentially out-of-control chaos of nature" (1996, p. 238).

Perhaps nowhere is this penchant for the mundane more evident than in the authorized treatments performed by rehabilitation therapists. Here, the predictable intervention constitutes what is publicly reportable and reimbursable. The dramatic, by contrast, constitutes an "underground practice" among therapists—what they sometimes do, and even sometimes cherish, but rarely publicly admit or defend (Mattingly & Fleming, 1994; Mattingly, 1998b). There will be no reports by Amy of tea parties or the fleeting appearance of a gracious and socially-engaged witch in the medical chart. In the public discourse of the rehabilitation clinic, the individual-ized, improvisational, and imaginative are always suppressed in the name of repeatable routines. Even physicians, who are themselves keenly aware that they must build trusting relationships with patients and families, and in this sense "individualize" certain aspects of their practice, protest when therapists do not follow strict routines in their treatment protocols.

In rehabilitation therapies (dominated by the physical-occupational-speech triad), routinization is accomplished through a focus on relearn-ing bodily skills that are very often treated as disconnected from a person and her life. However, rehabilitation has some special features that distin-guish it from many other clinical encounters. While patients are very often required to be passive within the hospital, to wait, to lie still, to render their bodies docile and inert, rehabilitation asks something quite different. Rehabilitative professionals demand active patients. Docility here takes the form of hard work, a daily struggle with one's body. And practitioners themselves are also active, assessing a patient's status, etiology, and prog-nosis by attending to bodies in motion, seeing what they can do, and by moving their own bodies in ways that facilitate the movements of their patients. When patients are in rehabilitation, they are involved in "doing therapies" where actions, often everyday actions, form the core of treat-ment (Mattingly, 1998b, 2000).

Though therapists are generally unwilling to report deviations from the routine, many therapists resist reducing their interventions in narrowly bio-mechanical terms, though their resistance may not take them far. Their rebellion is sometimes propelled by the patients, particularly in pediatrics. Children like Leia and Felicia tend to refuse to cooperate with painful or boring routines and many therapists are unwilling to treat a screaming, tantrum throwing or sullenly catatonic child for 45 minutes. Some therapists, like Amy, are also inspired by a vision of what constitutes effective practice which demands embedding routine exercises within imaginative activities—in other words, some kind of creative play.

Perhaps the most powerful impediment to the recognition and cultivation of healing dramas within the modern clinic has to do with the disconnection between what healers like Amy or Penny believe, in an almost private way, to be important for a given patient, and what they feel they can legitimately claim to know. Their claims to authoritative knowledge do not include the capacity to redirect treatment to tackle diagnostically diffuse emotional and behavioral problems of their patients, especially not when treatment looks, as Penny remarks dejectedly, like "just a social thing." Turf issues and a myriad of other institutional factors stand between these healers and their own "personal knowledge," to use Michael Polanyi's important term (1966). In such situations, Western biomedicine, with its particular claims to authoritative knowledge, not only undermines confidence in the embodied knowledge of sufferers (Jordon, 1993; Browner & Press, 1995; Sargent & Bascope, 1996) but also of the healers themselves. Yet the cultivation of healing dramas in which, for instance, Leia can participate in nurturing, or Felicia can cultivate her wit and charm, demand that healers draw upon their own embodied knowledge. Penny's understanding of the hopelessness one might feel being perpetually trapped in a cramped apartment with nothing but junk food and small children, fuels her drive to build a positive self-image in Felicia. To do so, she must also have the flexibility to follow leads provided by Felicia herself. Adhering to a strictly prescribed routine is antithetical to the kind of therapeutic attention demanded in creating such healing dramas.

CONCLUSION

Beneath the highly visible machinery of the modern clinic, with its elaborate technology, mind numbing routinization and cool dispassion, all sorts of other strange and even miraculous healing dramas may spring up, and in the most unlikely ways. Some of these are precipitated by patients or their families, some are even created in league with professionals themselves. In these narrative moments, recovery may not mean regaining faculties one once had, but it does mean reclaiming a body, discovering where and how movement is possible. In such moments, exercises and other therapeutic tasks emerge as healing dramas. These dramas may be hidden from professional view as Sacks relates in his own case. Or they may be discounted by professionals, not seen as fundamental to healing. Whether professionally recognized or ignored, these dramas share certain common features. They concern moments experienced by the participants as significant, time in which something is at stake. This "at stakeness" transforms mere experience, the forgettable everyday, to "an experience" with narrative form. In other writing, Mattingly (1994, 1998a) has used the construct "therapeutic emplotment" to designate those moments in which a dramatic figure is shaped in time itself. Healing, in a practice like occupational therapy at least, very often involves creating activities imaginatively rich enough to convey the moral that, despite a body lost, broken, or largely silent, there still exists a self worth making, worth struggling for. Morals are embodied in actions themselves and in the dramas that surround taking action when a body (and a self) is threatened. But not just any sort of action will do.

The clinical actions that create dramas, those with transformative and healing potential, must matter deeply to the patient. They must call to the body. Very often they are part of an old body knowledge, a powerfully, highly valued, ingrained, and tacit mode of being in the world. *Experience itself becomes the focus of attention for the patient.* The body may have its techniques, its practices, its efficiencies and breakdowns that can be neatly rendered and reasoned about in those mechanical metaphors that abound in rehabilitation. But in these moments, such qualities are taken up in the experience of movement itself, and movement toward something, movement for something, movement of no mere material matter but of one's very self.

Healing dramas within the world of rehabilitation have a public, socially constructed character. They are rather like improvisational plays involving multiple characters, each finding their parts and cuing one another about what ought to happen next. These dramas are very much created between therapists and patients, and family members as well, so that it is clear that significant experience is not something which is merely privately felt and intuited but something that exists in the public world. In depicting his own recovery from a leg injury, Sacks tells a story which insists on the centrality of drama to healing, where drama is understood in deeply phenomenological terms, an experience of the body, one where the body is vividly marked as the "seat" not only of experience but also of self identity. In these dramatic moments, the body is experienced in a different way. It is transformed from impediment and obstacle to a site of possibility. Experience takes the shape of an imaginary journey from illness to recovery, even if, as is often the case, it does not lead to any medical cure.

Healing dramas may be powerful, but they may also be fleeting, momentary bursts of life that cannot be sustained under a harsh clinical gaze. They are frail things, often created only to be interrupted, ignored, or undermined. It may sometimes be the case, as Van Blerkom argues in his study of "clown doctors," that "Western medical practitioners increasingly recognize the need to escape the limitations of a bioreductionist view of health and disease" (1995, p. 465). Among the rehabilitation therapists I have studied, however, I have not found an ability among practitioners to accommodate to different models of healing simultaneously or to see them as complimentary. Rather, I have witnessed a deep unease as practitioners initiate healing dramas that they then feel forced to relinquish when their treatment approach departs too visibly from authorized clinical care.

In this paper, I have offered an anatomy of two such moments of initiation and abandonment within the world of pediatric rehabilitation. The significance of the experiences created is fragile and easily lost not only because lived experience necessarily has a fleeting quality but because the cultural worlds in which these experiences occur do not authorize these kinds of healing dramas. They have no official status within clinic culture for they are not acknowledged as integral to healing. When Sacks's experiences of recovery are not shared by his healers, he improves anyway. He recovers both his leg and his life. As it turns out, his healing is not dependent upon his healers' recognition of the dramas of recovery. Felicia, Leia, and the other children in our studies are not so lucky. They are not blessed with the resources Sacks draws upon, and their injuries and illnesses are far more serious. Felicia and Leia do encounter healers who seem to recognize, at some level, that healing in the world of chronic illness and disability requires the creation of significant moments, those that reveal possible worlds and possible selves worth striving for. But the dramas of recovery we have explored in their cases, created in concert with the therapists themselves, are constructed within the confines of institutional worlds. Such worlds largely constrain these professionals' vision of their task. When healing dramas are not sufficiently prized, healing falters, or fails altogether. Sacks preserves and recreates his experience through his storytelling powers and his own practice as a physician. But it is less clear that Felicia and Leia will be able to emplot their lives such that these dramatic moments become episodes in a larger and longer lasting drama of recovery.

REFERENCES

Becker, G. (1994). Metaphors in disrupted lives: Infertility and cultural constructions of continuity. *Medical Anthropology Quarterly, 8,* 383–410.

Becker, G. (1997). *Disrupted lives: How people create meaning in a chaotic world.* Berkeley, CA: University of California Press.

Becker, G., & Kaufman, S. R. (1995). Managing an uncertain illness trajectory in old age: Patients' and physicians' view of stroke. *Medical Anthropology Quarterly, 9,* 165–187.

Briggs, C. (1996). The meaning of nonsense, the poetics of embodiment, and the production of power in Warao healing. In C. Laderman & M. Roseman (Eds.), *The performance of healing* (pp. 185–232). London: Routledge.

Brockmeier, J. (2002). Autobiographical remembering as cultural practice: Understanding the interplay between memory, self, and culture. *Culture & Psychology, 8,* 45–64.

Browner, C. H., & Press, N. A. (1995). The normalization of prenatal diagnostic screening. In F. D. Ginsburg & R. Rapp (Eds.), *Conceiving the New World Order: The politics of reproduction* (pp. 307–322). Berkeley, CA: University of California Press.

Bruner, J. (1986). *Actual minds, possible worlds.* Cambridge, MA: Harvard University Press.

Bruner, J. (1990). *Acts of meaning.* Cambridge, MA: Harvard University Press.

Bruner, J. (1991). The narrative construction of reality. *Critical Inquiry, 18,* 1–21.

Bülow, P. H. & Hydén, L.C. (2003). In dialogue with time: Identity and illness in narratives about chronic fatigue. *Narrative Inquiry, 13,* 71–97.

Cain, C. (1991). Personal stories: Identity acquisition and self-understanding in Alcoholics Anonymous. *Ethos, 19,* 210–253.

Carr, D. (1986). *Time, narrative, and history.* Bloomington: Indiana University Press.

Carr, D. (1997). Narrative and the real world: An argument for continuity. In L. P. Hinchman & S. Hinchman (Eds.), *Memory, identity, community: The idea of narrative in the human sciences* (pp. 7–25). New York: State University of New York Press.

Charon, R., & Montello, M. (Eds.). (2002). *Stories matter: The role of narrative in medical ethics.* London: Taylor and Francis.

Crites, S. (1997). The narrative quality of experience. In L. P. Hinchman & S. Hinchman (Eds.), *Memory, identity, community: The idea of narrative in the human sciences* (pp. 26–50), New York: State University of New York Press.

Csordas, T. J. (1994). Introduction: The body as representation and being-in-the-world. In T. J. Csordas (Ed.), *Embodiment and experience* (pp. 1–24). Cambridge, UK: Cambridge University Press.

Csordas, T. (1996). Imaginal performance and memory in ritual healing, In C. Laderman & M. Roseman (Eds.), *The performance of healing* (pp. 91–113). London: Routledge.

Danforth, L. (1989). *Firewalking and religious healing: The Ana Stenari of Greece and the American Firewalking Movement.* Princeton: Princeton University Press.

Davis-Floyd, R., & Davis, E. (1996). Intuition as authentic knowledge in midwifery and home birth. *Medical Anthropology Quarterly, 10,* 237–269.

Desjarlais, R. (1996). Presence. In C. Laderman & M. Roseman (Eds.), *The performance of healing* (pp. 143–164). London: Routledge.

Dilthey, W. (1989). Introduction to the human sciences. In R. A. Makkreel & F. Rodi (Eds.), *William Dithey: Selected works* (Vol. I, pp. 55–240). Princeton: Princeton University Press.

Frank, A. (1995). *The wounded storyteller: Body, illness, and ethics.* Chicago: University of Chicago Press.

Gadamer, H-G. (1975). *Truth and method.* New York: Seabury Press.

Gadamer, H-G. (1996). *The enigma of health: The art of healing in a scientific age.* Stanford: Stanford University Press

Garro, L. (2000). Cultural knowledge as resource in illness Narratives: remembering through accounts of illness. In C. Mattingly & L. Garro (Eds.), *Narrative and the cultural construction of illness and healing* (pp. 70–87). Berkeley, CA: University of California Press.

Good B., & Good, M-J. (1994). In the subjunctive mode: Epilepsy narratives in Turkey. *Social Science & Medicine, 36,*835–842.

Greenhalgh, T., & Hurwitz, B. (Eds.). (1998). *Narrative based medicine. Dialogue and discourse in clinical practice.* London: BMJ Books.

Hughes-Freeland, F. (1998). Introduction. In F. Hughes-Freeland (Ed.), *Ritual, performance, media* (pp. 1–28). London and New York: Routledge.

Hunter, K. (1991). *Doctor's stories: The narrative structure of medical knowledge.* Princeton: Princeton University Press.

Hydén, L. C. (1997). Illness and narrative. *Sociology of Health & Illness, 19,* 48–69.

Jackson, J. (1989). *Paths toward a clearing: Radical empiricism and ethnographic inquiry.* Bloomington: Indiana University Press.

Jordan, B. (1993). *Birth in four cultures: A cross cultural investigation of childbirth in Yucatan, Holland, Sweden and the United States* (4th ed.). Prospect Heights, IL: Waveland Press.

Kapferer, B. (1983). *A celebration of demons: Exorcism and the aesthetics of healing in Sri Lanka.* Bloomington: Indiana University Press.

Kapferer, B. (1986). Performance and the structuring of meaning and experience. In V. Turner & E. Bruner (Eds.), *The anthropology of experience* (pp. 188–203). Urbana, IL: University of Illinois Press.

Kendall, L. (1996). Initiating performance: The story of Chini, a Korean shaman. In C. Laderman & M. Roseman (Eds.), *The performance of healing* (pp. 17–58). London: Routledge.

Kirmayer, L. (2000). Broken narratives: Clinical encounters and the poetics of illness experience. In C. Mattingly & L. Garro (Eds.), *Narrative and the cultural construction of illness and healing* (pp. 153–180). Berkeley, CA: University of California Press.

Kleinman, A. (1988). The illness narratives: Suffering, healing, and the human condition. New York: Basic Books.

Laderman, C. (1996). The poetics of healing in Malay shamanistic performances. In C. Laderman & M. Roseman (Eds.), *The performance of healing* (pp. 115–147). London: Routledge.

MacIntyre, A. (1981). *After virtue: A study in moral theory.* South Bend, IN: University of Notre Dame Press.

Mattingly, C. (1994). The concept of therapeutic 'emplotment.' *Social Science and Medicine, 38,* 811–822.

Mattingly, C. (1998a). In search of the good: Narrative reasoning in clinical practice. *Medical Anthropology Quarterly, 12,* 273–297.

Mattingly, C. (1998b). *Healing dramas and clinical plots: The narrative structure of experience.* Cambridge, UK: Cambridge University Press.

Mattingly, C. (2000). Emergent narratives. In C. Mattingly & L. Garro (Eds.), *Narrative and the cultural construction of illness and healing* (pp. 181–211). Berkeley, CA: University of California Press.

Mattingly, C., & Fleming, M. (1994). *Clinical reasoning: Forms of inquiry in therapeutic practice.* Philadelphia: F.A. Davis.

Medved, M. I., & Brockmeier, J. (2004). Making sense of traumatic experiences: Telling your life with Fragile X syndrome. *Qualitative Health Research, 14,* 741–759.

Monks, J. (2000). Talk as social suffering: Narratives of talk in medical settings. *Anthropology & Medicine, 7,* 15–38.

Morris, D. (1998). *Illness and culture in the postmodern age.* Berkeley, CA: University of California Press.

Olafson, F. (1979). *The dialectic of action: Philosophical interpretation of history and the humanities.* Chicago: University of Chicago Press.

Polanyi, M. (1966). *The tacit dimension.* Garden City, NY: Doubleday.

Polkinghorne, D. E. (1988). *Narrative knowing and the human sciences.* Albany, NY: State University of New York.

Rhodes, L. (1993). The shape of action. In S. Lindenbaum & M. Lock (Eds.), *Knowledge, power and practice* (pp. 129–144). Berkeley, CA: University of California Press.

Ricoeur, P. (1983). *Time and narrative, Vol. I* (K. McLaughlin & De. Pallauer, trans.). Chicago: University of Chicago Press.

Ricoeur, P. (1984). *Time and narrative, Vol. 2* (K. McLaughlin & De. Pallauer, trans.). Chicago: University of Chicago Press.

Sacks, Oliver (1987). *A leg to stand on.* New York: Summit Books.

Sargent, C., & Bascope, G. (1996). Ways of knowing about birth in three cultures. *Medical Anthropology Quarterly, 10,* 213–236.

Schechner, R. (1990). Magnitudes of performance. In R. Schechner & A. Willa (Eds.), *By means of performance: Intercultural studies of theatre and ritual* (pp. 19–49). Cambridge, UK: Cambridge University Press.

Schieffelin, E. (1996). On failure and performance: Throwing the medium out of the seance. In C. Laderman & M. Roseman, (Eds.), *The performance of healing* (pp. 59–89). London: Routledge.

Stern, D. N. (1994). One way to build a clinically relevant baby. *Infant Mental Health Journal, 15,* 9–25.

Stern, D. N. (1995). *The motherhood constellation.* New York: Basic Books.

Stoller, P. (1989). *The taste of ethnographic things: The senses of anthropology.* Philadelphia: University of Pennsylvania Press.

Stoller, P. (1996). Sounds and things: Pulsations of power in Songhay. In C. Laderman & M. Roseman (Eds.), *The performance of healing* (pp. 165–184). London: Routledge.

Stoller, P. (1997). *Sensuous scholarship.* Philadelphia: University of Pennsylvania Press.

Tambiah, S. (1985). Culture, thought and social action: An anthropological perspective. Cambridge, UK: Cambridge University Press.

Turner, E. (1992). *Experiencing ritual: A new interpretation of African healing.* Philadelphia: University of Pennsylvania Press.

Turner, V. (1969). *The ritual process: Structure and anti-structure.* Chicago: Aldine.

Turner, V. (1986a). *The anthropology of performance.* New York: PAJ Publications.

Turner, V. (1986b). Dewey, Dilthey, and drama: An essay in the anthropology of experience. In V. Turner & E. M. Bruner, (Eds.), *The anthropology of experience* (pp. 33–44). Chicago: University of Illinois Press.

Van Blerkom, L. M. (1995). Clown doctors: Shaman healers of Western medicine. *Medical Anthropology Quarterly, 9,* 462–475.

Wikan, U. (2000). With life in one's lap: The story of an eye/I (or two). In C. Mattingly & L. Garro (Eds.), *Narrative and the cultural construction of illness and healing* (pp. 212–236). Berkeley, CA: University of California Press.

6 Globally Distributed Silences, and Broken Narratives About HIV

Georg Drakos

How do silences about HIV shape the conditions for what it is like to live with HIV (and die of) the disease? How are silences used to create meaning and experiences? Many people with HIV keep silent about the disease in many contexts. The most obvious reason surely is that the disease seems to be able to give rise to social stigmatization all over the world. At the start of 2005, Nelson Mandela announced that his son had died of AIDS. In his television appearance he emphasized the importance of talking openly about the disease, thereby breaking the silence that is so often caused by shame and fear of stigmatization. In South Africa HIV/AIDS was not recognized as a serious national problem until the end of the 1990s. The current president, Thabo Mbeki, has become known to the world for not accepting the medical explanation for what causes AIDS and how the disease should be treated. He has instead stubbornly held up poverty as crucial for the development of the epidemic, and seemed not to agree with the medical understanding of the epidemic. This and other statements in connection with the AIDS conference in Durban in 2000 led a number of delegates at the conference, which had the motto "Breaking the silence," to issue a declaration that AIDS is caused by HIV.

How the motto of the conference is interpreted and evaluated depends on which silences the appeal is addressed to. Was it the silence of the uneducated African that had to be broken? Was it the authorities' attempts to silence the association between HIV and AIDS that was to be replaced by plain language? Was it the smoke screens surrounding the profit interests of the pharmaceutical industry that had to be dispersed? Or was there a vision that the thundering of the drums that accompanied the opening of the AIDS conference in Durban would be heard all the way to those countries that had succeeded in controlling the HIV epidemic within their own borders, to prevent their media and authorities from silencing the continued human catastrophe in the poor world?

These questions can't be answered without being contextualized. This is also my way to approach silences. More exactly I approach silences about HIV by examining their narrative contexts, in what ways silences are linked to narratives. Among all kinds of silences, certainly there are those which are not loaded with meaning. But these I have in mind often carry the most loaded knowledge. I am concerned of silences kept on purpose, either personally intended silences or silences officially distributed by authorities. With this point of departure I conceptualize silences in terms of "broken narratives," a metaphor that links narratives with silences and thereby provides a tool for analyzing silences empirically.

I will base my examination of broken narratives about HIV on a study of what it is like to live as next of kin to a person with HIV/AIDS in Sweden and Greece (Drakos, 2005, 2006). In other words, in parts of the world and at a point in time where modern HIV treatment is available to everyone who needs it. One of my most powerful experiences in the field is that people with HIV and their nearest keep silent about the disease in many contexts.

This linkage between narratives and silences is a property that could describe all narration if we regard narrative and silence as two sides of the same coin. It is then in the nature of narration that every narrative constitutes one kind of reality and simultaneously silences others and, that all narratives carry broken narratives in some sense. This makes every narrative a stance or a negotiation about what reality is like. It is above all from this point of view that I have taken an interest in broken narratives to do with HIV.

Both silences and narratives act on different levels. They are globally and locally distributed, and in turn they shape personal conditions for how it is like to live with HIV. The observation of the intended use of silences is by no means new. Almost a century ago, Georg Simmel described secrecy as a cultural practice in everyday life, through which groups and subgroups form and regulate their communication with the world (Simmel, 1999; Bendix, 2003). We later encounter the perspective in Erving Goffman's (1959) inter-action theory with the focus on the theatricality of everyday life, which of necessity includes a concealed, secret domain behind the stage. How we protect our private sphere from being publicly visible varies in different arenas and is associated with social and cultural practices at different levels, from interaction between individuals to the exercise of authority. (I have previously treated the interaction between these levels in my description of strategies for secretiveness among people with leprosy in today's Greece [Drakos 1997, pp. 106ff].)

The silence in the mass media in Sweden and Greece, after it became possible there and in much of Europe to curb the HIV epidemic with modern medicines, seems like an echo of the paradoxes of the modern social project. As Charles Briggs and Clara Mantini-Briggs (2003, p. 327) has been pointed out in a study of the epidemic of cholera that broke out in Venezuela in 1992–1993, the world that claims to uphold democracy and equality has, to an extent never seen before, laid the foundation for a hierarchization and exclusion of weak groups. What distinguishes poor from rich populations, modern societies from underdeveloped ones, is in large measure a matter of the unequal availability of medicines, public health, and hygiene, a fundamental inequality to which the development in the rich countries has contributed instead of eliminating it. The shared feature of leprosy, cholera, HIV/AIDS, and other terrifying epidemics, is that they generate globally and locally distributed silences that shape the conditions for what it is like to live with (and die of) the diseases. It seems to me that those silences reinforce inequality in regard to health. It also seems to me that breaking the silence about HIV for an individual can get very diverse effects.

In the following I will examine how narratives and silences about HIV shape the conditions for living with the disease and being a member of a Greek family where a person has HIV. With this example I want to test the usefulness of the concept of broken narratives, which does not concern people's inability to transform experiences into narrative form here. Broken narratives about HIV are instead seen as an expression of the way people in certain situations feel prevented from speaking openly about their own or relatives' experiences of the disease. I will approach broken narratives as a phenomenon arising in the tension between one's own or other people's demands for silences and the desire to tell stories. The three parts of the article deal with three observations of the relationship between narratives and silences. The first confirms Simmel's statement that secrecy is an everyday practice for steering communication with the rest of the world. The second observation is that people's narratives and secrecy are embodied practices. The reason for this is that narrators always "are their body," and through narratives or silences about HIV expose or conceal the state of their own bodies. The third observation is that narratives and silences are a cultural practice and can therefore shed light on the significance of cultural differences for what it is like to be a relative of a person with HIV.

BROKEN NARRATIVES—EVERYDAY PRACTICES

The Greek family to which I will refer consists of the parents and their two grown-up children. The children, whom I call Aris and Theodora, grew up in a little village in southern Greece but were living in Athens when I met them. (Apart from using pseudonyms I have changed some details to protect the family's integrity.) The parents and some of their relatives still live in the village. Theodora had HIV, probably infected by the man with whom she was living at the end of the 1980s. They both received their diagnoses of HIV in 1992. The man, whom I call Petros, developed AIDS and died a few years later. Theodora, however, had not suffered from any sequelae, probably as a result of the medical treatment she underwent.

Like many other people with HIV, Theodora was anxious to keep control of who was to know about her diagnosis. This need was ignored, however, as soon as she learned of the diagnosis because the results of the test were leaked to several of her relatives. The breach of secrecy meant that Theodora's relatives received the information before she did herself, and that she did not know, and still does not, who was informed that she had

HIV. Apart from Petros and her parents, she had not spoken openly about her disease until a few months before I met her at the end of March 2001. It was only then that she and her brother Aris had broken a long mutual silence about her HIV infection and she told the truth about the real disease that had caused Petros's death. The conversations with Aris, Theodora, and later with their mother show how well integrated broken narratives can be in people's daily lives and how they sometimes threaten to break out and involuntarily change the conditions for their communication with the outside world.

I came into contact with Theodora through a support organization in Athens. I had been invited to take part in a conversation group consisting of persons with HIV, their next of kin, and some volunteers. Who belonged to which category was one of the personal details about which the group deliberately did not speak openly. I was able to inform them about my ongoing research project and my interest in interviewing people with HIV and their next of kin or relatives. Theodora was one of those who approached me after the conversation group ended to say that she would be willing to take part in interviews. When I met her a couple of days later, the broken narrative about her experiences of HIV was the subject that she spontaneously brought up first. I had told her a little about my study and its orientation, and she had asked me how many similar studies about HIV/AIDS were being conducted at Greek institutions. I mentioned what I knew about the research being done at the National School of Public Health in Athens, which led Theodora to begin talking about herself as follows (for transcription conventions, see note at the end):

> Theodora: For me anyway, this is the first time that I'm talking abut this subject [yes] and I really haven't spoken this openly about it with anybody, just with a doctor [¿with a doctor] Mm.
> Georg: And with your brother?
> Theodora: Everyone else, my parents, my brother, my friends, my cousins, heard about it from elsewhere.
> Georg: From elsewhere! [yes] How did that happen?
> Theodora: It was presumably spread at the hospital where I was, not by the doctor but by others around him. It was told to some acquaintance, who told somebody else and then everybody found out about it. I can say that I was the last to learn. Everybody knew about it, my parents knew about it and my doctor told me last.

I was surprised and shaken by her account of something which, at least in the Swedish health service, would have been regarded as a flagrant breach of confidentiality. I later found out that this was the case in Greece as well. One difference was perhaps due to the circumstance that more relatives tend to be physically present around patients in Greece than in Sweden, and that confidentiality may therefore be harder to maintain. But just as in Swedish health care, the patient is the first to hear the diagnosis and can then decide whether other people should be told about it. There may possibly be differences in practice between the countries in certain other serious diagnoses. Several of my Greek colleagues have suggested, with some exaggeration, that HIV and cancer generate opposite flows of information. Whereas a HIV patient receives his or her diagnosis and then keeps it secret, only the relatives are told when a person has contracted cancer. I myself have witnessed the latter on a couple of occasions. The fact that Theodora began by describing how she received her diagnosis and not how she became infected made me ask why she did so. She then told me that she had had a sexual relationship.

> Theodora: Okay, I had a sexual relationship then. I had had a relation-
> ship since '89, for roughly 3 years. The only thing I can say, but
> without claiming to be sure, is that my boyfriend had used some
> substance before, not when we were together, before that.
> Georg: You mean drugs?
> Theodora: Yes, he had had an intensive erotic life. I don't know exactly
> how important that was.

From her account I drew the conclusion that she had been infected by her partner, but I have subsequently realized that I did not really have any evidence as to how the virus had reached her. But Theodora told me that she had been with one or at most two men before she met the man that I later understood was Petros. Since she began the cited sequence by speaking of her relationship in the past tense, I also drew the conclusion that it had ended.

> Georg: Don't you have any contact with him now?
> Theodora: He's gone now, he's away.
> Georg: Is he dead?
> Theodora: Yes.
> Georg: Of what?
> Theodora: Of this. Of, okay, of swollen lymphatic glands for 2 years. We
> were together and . .
> Georg: Had you been together a long time?
> Theodora: For one period we weren't, but most of the time we were
> together. And I was there during the phase of a year or a year and
> a half when he was in hospital getting medical treatment. I saw
> Petros languish away.
> Georg: It seems as if you've been through a lot, I understand that.
> Theodora: It was very hard for me. And I still don't think I've taken it in
> that he's gone. I, I tell myself that he's better off where he is. In the
> last phase he was very poorly, and where he is now he's better off.
> That's what I say [hm mm]. And now roughly 2 years have passed
> since he passed away. And my parents were against the relation-
> ship from the beginning. They were negative about the relationship
> because they knew about Petros. And when they learned about

this too it was obvious that he was to blame and okay, we had a lot of problems. In other words, threats that they would, you know, shoot him, things like that. But, with the exception of a period when we weren't together because he had gone away to work, to Ioannina, we were apart for about a year and a half. Otherwise we were together the whole time right up to the end.

This was how Theodora described her relationship with Petros in our conversation. Her clarification "He's dead now, he's away" to my question whether they were in contact with each other sounded to my ears as if she wanted to say that death had not separated them forever, that he was now "away," roughly as when he had been away working, not that he was forever dead and buried. Immediately after the above she went on:

> Theodora: And I didn't think I would be able. .
>
> I still can't . .
>
> There are times when I can't believe it. I tell myself that he's just gone away, somewhere else [hm]
>
> And they have him there, at a memorial place, where I haven't been a single time. I can't go there. And I don't know if I'll ever be able to, since he's not there for me. I can't accept that the man I was together with is there. That's how it is
>
> (laughs sadly) That's how it is.

Theodora gave me a powerful impression of not being willing or able to reconcile herself with Petros's death. At the same time, in the passage of our conversation that I have just quoted she had said that her parents had never accepted her relationship with Petros and that they had become increasingly unforgiving after they had drawn the conclusion that he had infected her with HIV. These two interpretations of the reality of the disease, Theodora's loss of the man she loved, and the parents' interpretation that Petros was to blame for their daughter's disease, are obviously difficult to reconcile. But the conflict between the story one can presume that the parents would choose to tell about Petros and the story that Theodora had told puts the protracted silence between her and Aris about the disease into perspective. A couple of minutes after the sequence just quoted, Theodora returned to this subject when describing her move to Athens and her current life situation.

> Theodora: My brother came here to work and/
> Georg: Just so that I can understand—you shared a home, did you?
> Theodora: Yes, and we still live together [I understand]. And our parents are down in the village. We are from Chorio, which is near Patras.
> Georg: Have you any other brothers or sisters?

> **Theodora:** No, there's just the two of us. And me and my brother spoke for the first time to each other this year about it, even though he knew. . I knew that he knew about it, but I didn't want us to talk about it. I didn't want us to be grieved by it [hm hm]
>
> That was stupid, of course. You know, when we talked with each other it did us both good. But we waited a bit with that [¿But] But (smiles knowingly) we waited a bit with that.

Theodora's explanation for having waited for over 7 years to tell Aris openly about her HIV infection—although she knew all the time that he was already informed—raises new questions. How had she envisaged the situation that would have arisen if she had spoken out? If we look at her description of her parents' reactions to the news that she had HIV, a hypothesis that easily comes to mind is that she wanted to avoid a similar situation between her and her brother. By preventing Aris from bringing up the subject through her own silence, she avoided exposing herself to the risk that he, like the parents, would respond with arguments about Petros as a threat to the family's reputation. Even if, in retrospect, she had been able to see that Aris had not reacted this way, many examples from older and more recent Greek ethnography show that the expected complementarity in the roles of family members can generate such stances and positions (see, e.g., Campbell, 1976, p. 157, 268ff; Friedl, 1962, pp. 84ff, 1986, pp. 42ff; Herzfeld, 1991, pp. 79ff).

On an individual level, the requirement to keep different worlds separate can be due to various factors. It is far from unique that people with HIV avoid informing one or more members of their own family, relatives, or other people close to them. In Theodora's family the breach of confidentiality in connection with the HIV test gave rise to a kind of double life, which became particularly difficult for her and her brother to handle, since they were living together. The result was that they said less and less to each other, their exchanges becoming devoid of anything meaningful. This was the picture painted for me by Aris, whom I interviewed a few days after my talk with Theodora. From that point of view, their mutual demand for silence became a kind of taboo, a prohibition on the type of narratives that could be the consequence of one of them bringing up the subject of HIV/AIDS. I use the word taboo because it also invokes ideas about the requirement to separate certain categories and states in human interaction and prevent inappropriate boundary transgressions. This prohibition, which was based on unspoken agreements in the siblings' interaction, had a strength that made both Theodora and her brother incapable of exchanging narratives and creating meaning around the disease that was affecting Theodora physically, mentally, and socially, but which also intervened in her brother's life.

In the interview Aris emphasized his satisfaction that the silence about his sister's HIV infection was finally broken in their interaction. In the narrative to which our conversation gave rise, the event when the silence was broken stands out as a distinct turning point in his relationship to his sister. He explained that he and Theodora had never been really close to each other, but that their conversations with each other, as a consequence of the mutual silence about her HIV diagnosis, had been reduced to greetings or routine phrases and answers about practical matters in everyday life. This silence had become increasingly unbearable for him. In retrospect it is not difficult to envisage the social dynamics that surrounded the sibling's mutual silence, and their exchanges contained countless forms of nonnarrative communication which never developed into narratives. Both siblings were aware that several of their relatives knew about the HIV diagnosis. A similar comment is made by Laurence J. Kirmayer (2000, p. 175) about communication in a clinical context; he points out that broken narratives can also draw attention to other voices that speak through those who are present. Asking ourselves questions about broken narratives can moreover mean that we become attentive to potential narratives which are never told, only hinted at or perhaps able to be told only in a particular situation.

I heard one such narrative in my second interview with Aris, when we sketched his family's genealogical diagram together (cf. Stylianoudi, 1996). I used the method to gain insight into how people connect difficult or bewildering events in the present with the history of the family. The narrative that was triggered as we drew Aris's genealogical diagram was to give Theodora's HIV infection a dramatic new meaning. With a certain degree of pride, he told how their family had long been well known far beyond their own village. He took as an example the fact that a fellow passenger on the bus trip home to the village once had shown that he knew the family when Aris introduced himself. This shed an explanatory light on the fact that, at our first meeting of the support organization together with this sister, he had wanted to know whether the surnames of my interviewees would be published in the study. The family name was known through an almost mythical narrative about the origin of the family.

Briefly, it was about the abduction of a woman that resulted in the marriage of his paternal grandparents. He described his grandfather as the head of the family, and I noted that Aris and Theodora were named after their grandparents, whose names also recurred elsewhere in the family diagram. Aris began the story by relating how the man who would later become his grandfather had asked for the hand of a woman in a village on the other side of the river. He was refused and the woman was instead betrothed to a rival suitor. But on the day when she was to be married, the grandfather appeared at the church, on horseback in full regalia, and accompanied by two men. He seized the bride and rode off with her into the mountains. The woman's relatives swore that a curse would strike his family for all time. His life together with the woman lasted just 5 years, for he was fighting in the Greek civil war and was brutally executed by his enemies. Aris said that he remembered his relatives searching the mountains for his remains as late as the 1980s, without result. He hinted that the story of his grandfather's fate had had a negative influence on the family, that it has been afflicted by discord and internal conflicts. According to Aris, the stories about how he stole the bride and later died in the civil war are well known and have even become the stuff of ballads. Marriage by abduction is a recurrent theme in Greek ethnography in rural contexts (see, e.g., Campbell, 1976, pp. 124ff; Herzfeld, 1988, pp. 20, 25, 52, 152, 162, 180, 288f; Seremetakis, 1991, p. 38).

While silences separate different realities, narratives bind them together. This is one reason why the narrative about Theodora's disease could take on a new meaning if it is linked to the abduction of the bride by Aris's grandfather. The story of the abduction can therefore provide yet another contextual explanation for the family's earnest desire to keep silent in the village about what had happened to Theodora. It is conceivable that the family was thereby protecting itself against being inscribed in the previous generation's narrative about the abduction and the curses pronounced on Aris's grandfather and his descendants. If this happened, the infection that had struck Theodora and led to the death of her lover could be transformed into the evil destiny of the family. This transformation, in other words, could be triggered by an event in the family's distant past (the abduction) being brought to life in connection with a serious event in the present (Theodora's HIV infection) and in connection with this current event seems to be active as a broken narrative in the family's everyday practice.

BROKEN NARRATIVES—EMBODIED PRACTICES

The statement that narratives and silences shape the conditions for what it is like to live with HIV/AIDS is based on the fact that we use narratives to interpret how diseases arise, not just in the body but also in life and in society. Narratives establish the terms for their own interpretation. Another condition of interpretation shapes a person's own body as a medium and is a point of departure for narration (Frank, 1997). If we regard the human body in a phenomenological sense as a lived relation to the world, not as a static object, every human action has its origin in the body. We "are" our bodies, both when we talk and when we keep silent. Telling stories and relating to narratives and silences in the world around us is an embodied practice. While many people with HIV and their relatives find a good balance in deciding in consensus whom they will confide in and whom they will not inform, and do not find this particularly difficult, others can feel that the demand to observe silence is an enforced and frustrating burden. If we take into consideration the fact that HIV/AIDS seems to be able to give rise to social stigmatization all over the world, the silences about the disease can be both indicators of social suffering and instrumental means to avoid suffering. When viewed in this way, silences like suffering are embodied responses to certain situations.

Theodora's family is an example of how the silences about the disease are a response to complex situations which can be interpreted in different ways by different family members. The most obvious differences are those between Theodora's and the parents' interpretations of the situation that requires silence about her HIV infection. In that situation her relationship with Petros was a watershed. In her account, Theodora painted a clear picture of the conflict to which her relationship with Petros had given rise in her parental home. For herself, Petros represented all the good things she lacked in her parents. For the parents, Petros represented all the evil that threatened to damage the family. Theodora's account delineates the two contradictory narratives about Petros. One stresses his human qualities and his potential to contribute to the life together that Theodora valued. The other narrative highlights his divorce and previous use of drugs. Theodora said that this rumor had spread through the village, and that the problems had mounted from the day it reached her parents.

The parents threatened that Theodora would have to leave home if she insisted on carrying on the relationship. The threat must be partly understood in the light of a social context where the influence of the collective is expected to be more important than that of the individual. From the parents' point of view at least, one can envisage that Petros's bad reputation not only made him an undesirable candidate to marry their daughter and threatened the family's good name. It is also likely that Theodora's neglect of the family's reputation through her choice of Petros could be regarded by people other than her parents as a disloyal act and a breach of norms. Being forced to leave home can thus be viewed as a concrete solution to the problem, as a way to put her unacceptable relationship out of sight of neighbours and protect the family's collective body. Theodora seemed to reflect on this situation when, after my follow-up question, she continued her narrative.

Georg: You left?

Theodora: I tried to balance it all, but I don't know, perhaps it was better for me to leave because they have never accepted the relationship. Not even in the end did they accept my relationship with Petros, who I'd been with for about 10 years.

Georg: I can imagine you feel some bitterness with your parents.

Theodora: Yes, a lot. It's calmed down a bit now. Perhaps because Petros has died and there's nothing to quarrel about. But right up until the day Petros passed away and I visited his home. . My parents didn't come with me, of course, and they didn't understand why I went there, to the home of the person I'd been together with for 10 years! For them. . For my father, who told me I ought not to go there. That makes me very bitter.

In the cited sequence Theodora emphasizes her parents' implacable attitude to her relationship with Petros. The mere fact that Petros is now dead and that the relationship has ceased seems to have had the result that her parents have calmed down. This interpretation is reinforced by Theodora's continued and repeated narrative about her bitterness about their failure even to accept his life in connection with his burial, which paradoxically also seems to have made it more difficult for Theodora to accept his death. Had the parents' attempt to ignore the significance of their relationship prevented her from mourning his death publicly? In the midst of her lone grief, Theodora expressed an anger that still did not give her peace about Petros's death. In the next breath she described this anger:

> **Theodora:** I exploded, I accused them of many things during that period. Okay, it was probably unfair, but I had a heavy weight inside me, I was badly wounded emotionally [I understand]. I mean, I couldn't understand how they could care more about people, outsiders, than about me and my wishes. For they didn't want me to be with Petros, for fear of what people would say. What would they say about me being with a man like that? And they never felt what I felt. That hurt me a lot. A lot.
>
> And I went to visit Petros in hospital, when he was there. And my mother said to me: "Be careful nobody sees you!" Not: "How is Petros, how is he doing?" "Don't let anybody see you so that it gets out in the village!"

Both Aris's and Theodora's narratives about their experiences of living with a family member with HIV seemed to reproduce a voice that made their own family background resound. Both described themselves and each other as taciturn, claiming that this was a kind of family characteristic. When I later interviewed their mother in Athens she revealed other aspects of the family context which were significant for the lack of intimacy in the home. The mother, whom I call Panayota, was initially very hesitant about the conversation being recorded, and like Aris she referred to the fact that their name was well known. She described the family as taciturn, but she herself was talkative. She almost overflowed with her own narratives and seemed a little surprised at her own desire to tell stories. My lasting impression of the conversation was also her grief that Theodora had been infected by HIV. Most of all, however, she concentrated on the fact that she had not been able to give close support to her daughter, neither before nor now, 10 years after Theodora had received her diagnosis. She herself linked her inadequacy to external circumstances of their family life. Some way into the conversation, when I asked her to tell me about her own life, she first gave the following summary of the negative development of the family's life together.

Panayota: I was also born in the same county (as her husband). There were five children in our family, four girls and a boy. I'm the oldest. We were very happy with our two children, my mother was very pleased with me.

My husband was very good but another thing was that I had ended up in a fatherless family and my husband had to be like a father for both his older and his younger brothers and sisters in the home. And that was bad for us. My husband and I did not have a close relationship, like saying "let's do this or that today!" We didn't talk to each other at all, we always had people at home. Always packed with guests. All those from here and all those from outside. Up to 17–18 people, I had over ten people at home. And for a neighbour I had a sister-in-law and she didn't take care of a single one. And all this knocked me out. Financially too. We couldn't manage without working all summer. And we've been ruined financially.

Georg: So you had a lot of people in the family, [yes, a lot of people] in the home?

Panayota: Yes, lots of brothers and sisters. Together there were six from the village. There were two brothers in the same village. The one who was our neighbour, he didn't open the door to say: "Come on, dear brother—how will they have room to sleep? How can you have so many around the table?" And this made me very tired.

The situation she described was the major holidays, above all Easter, when the home became a gathering place for all the relatives. Having married into a "fatherless" family (as a consequence of the death of her husband's father in the civil war) was an important reason, she indicated, why her husband, and thereby also she herself, had ready-made roles to fill. That is how I interpret the narrative cited above in relation to the entire conversation in which she often returned to the family's dilemma, that the house was always full of relatives in leisure time and at holidays. Relatives took up too much space for the family's own economy and restricted the scope of their private lives. During the interview she revealed her tiredness by lying stretched out on the sofa opposite me, with a support collar to rest her back and neck. She also described how a gender regime dictated the division of labor in the home and the distribution of responsibility. When I asked if she could not have referred to her health problems in order to avoid having to do all the cooking and providing accommodation at the big holidays, she answered by quoting her husband:

Panayota: My husband wouldn't let me. It's years since I've. . He didn't even let me rest when I was like this. "Now when my brothers and sisters are coming, you're sick now? As soon as they leave you'll get well!" It's from all the work that my back, my legs, and my neck are ruined. Now when I lie down I notice that it gets better. I try, but I can't. That they come for Easter, that nine people gather in one house, that's a lot [sure, it's a lot]. And they come from Thursday, Friday until/

Georg: Do they all sleep in your home?

Panayota: Yes of course, but that's not the bad thing. That's why I'm telling you: She (a sister-in-law), the other woman had her life and just her own children to look after and has a closer relationship to her children. Me and my children are far from each other and that worries me a lot. The other day they (the sister-in-law's family) got up in the morning, I was upset that they didn't ask me and my daughter to come with them. They didn't need to cook or do anything. They went on a little excursion. "Where shall we eat?" And I'm under all this pressure.

With her body marked by overstrain, Panayota seemed bitter at having had to pay a high price without getting anything in return. As in the last quotation, she talked about having lost a close relationship to her children, as a consequence of large investments in the family's good name. Yet while Panayota complained of her predicament, with her narrative she established a kind of moral redress, having maintained the traditions of hospitality and other criteria for the family's reputation. She pointed out with satisfaction that Theodora took the same responsibility and declared that she had inherited this from her father who had in turn inherited it from his father, and she quoted her mother-in-law:

Panayota: "Like your father," my mother-in-law said to him (Panayota's husband). And to Theodora she said "you're like your father too, your hand is always open." If she has anything, she gives it away. And as small as she was when my mother-in-law looked after my children and my sister-in-law's children, she couldn't have a closed hand. If she had a bit of bread, they had to take it from her. But the other children weren't like that. That is hereditary.

Panayota returned several times to different meanings of the paternal heritage. When I revealed to her that I knew the story of her father-in-law, she replied: "Yes, he stole my mother-in-law" and told me how the abduction had come about.

Panayota: My father-in-law had asked for my mother-in-law's hand, and her family had answered, "We're not giving her in marriage, she's too young." After a short time she was engaged to another man and they were going to be married. And then, you know, they came on horses to take the bride up in the mountains where they hung out. And I remember my father-in-law saying, "You didn't give her to me. You gave her to a man who is below me!"

And at the same moment that the bridegroom goes to fetch the bride, they (the men) come out in front of them and take the bride who was about to be married. And then comes my father-in-law with his brothers, with some. . and they seize the bride. But the judge sided with my father-in-law, he knew the parents. He grabbed my mother-in-law and the others had to go home without a bride. But they pronounced many curses. Curses, you know? [yes, yes] evil [¿In what way] His (the bridegroom's) mother said to him, "It would have been better if you had shot them all instead of coming back without a bride!" That they should have been shot. Instead of having succeeded in their exploit.

The legacy of the abduction was linked to the family's name, and according to Panayota it still lived on as a hatred against the family among some people in the older generation. She also told about the sequel to the abduction in the form of two negative outcomes. One was the enforced marriage and the other was the man's early death in the Greek civil war. But she evaluated the events in these two spheres in different ways. On the one hand, she described her husband's father as a hero and martyr in the civil war, while she described his role in the enforced marriage as the opposite. When I asked her if her mother-in-law had perhaps had a secret love affair with the man who abducted her, she answered:

Panayota: They didn't reckon with that then. She didn't reckon with that. Nor being happy. They didn't bother about that. But we (Panayota and her husband) didn't feel any happiness either. And those who gather (in her home at holidays) don't ask us, "Do these people have room to talk to each other, to do things together, to go somewhere, to come to us, to bring the children?" That we too could bring the children, that we could dress our children, that they too could go somewhere. Huh, we went nowhere. They always got in first: "We're coming." We haven't been able to say no.

In this way she brought the story of the abduction back to her own family situation and linked her physical and social suffering both to the family's past and to its current situation. A dilemma in connection with the origin of the family was linked to a dilemma for the family's continued existence. This dilemma could be developed into an existential conflict if Theodora's disease was associated with her grandfather's abduction of his bride. The link between these two events could trigger a new narrative about a new and even more devastating abduction, at least if the narrative was told by a voice that wanted to harm the family. From this interpretative perspective, everyone who knew about Theodora's HIV diagnosis, but did not say a word about it, helped to protect her and the family, and perhaps themselves as close relatives, against the risk of being stigmatized. In this respect, the broken narrative about Theodora's

HIV diagnosis exists and is kept broken as an embodied response by everyone who helps to maintain the silence.

BROKEN NARRATIVES—CULTURAL PRACTICES

If by culture we mean a shared awareness which people reproduce and change by communicating with each other, then cultural differences and boundaries are seen on many levels and between different groups of people. Cultural differences not infrequently cut right across what might be perceived as a shared culture. I therefore regard culture as constructed and situationally formed in temporal, spatial, and social respects. This does not make cultural differences less real or less important. But the significance of cultural differences for what it is like to be a relative of a person with HIV also varies individually between people who in many respects share the same culture. It is not until differences are made visible that culture takes on meaning for people with HIV and their families. The silence about HIV has a global scope which conceals the lack of equality in health and is an expression of the force of modernization and the distribution of power in the world (Briggs & Mantini-Briggs, 2003, p. 198). This inequality gives openness and closedness different meanings in different parts of the world.

In the Swedish debate about HIV/AIDS, people have become accustomed to the fact that closedness is associated with ill health while openness is associated with a positive, healthier attitude. When accidents occur crisis groups are set up. For sick people and their relatives, groups are often organized where the members discuss their experiences together. In preventive work with HIV geared to men who have sex with men, the recommendation, at least from the gay movement, is often a secure sexual identity as an important means and end. The exhortation *"Come Out"* (*Kom Ut*), which is the characteristic title of the magazine of the Swedish federation for lesbian, gay, bisexual, and transgender rights (RFSL), advocates openness about sexuality and associates silence about one's own sexuality with insecurity. This exhortation is not particularly original or divergent in the Swedish public debate as a whole. In fact, it follows a dominant voice and uses a general narrative which connects openness and personal narration with positive self-esteem and well-being, or in a word: health.

There are countless examples of how this discourse has generated narratives in various fields. "Sex and personal relationships" (*"Sex och samlevnad"*) has been a central topic of health information in Sweden in recent decades, resulting, among other things, in extensive activity to improve sex education in schools and to prevent abortions. Long before this, as the ethnologist Maria Bäckman (2003, pp. 50ff) has pointed out, work for public health in Sweden was sustained by the idea of popular enlightenment, the belief in dialogue, and the idea that health can be created, planned, and taught, which is one reason why Sweden was first in the world in 1955 to have compulsory sex education in schools. (This is a basic idea in Western modernity that has been applied differently in different countries.) Parenthood and childbirth also have a long tradition of education in Sweden, through parents' groups, although this has not meant an unconditional dialogue with future parents. The ethnologist Susanne Nylund Skog (2002, p. 51) points out that dominant genres have been developed for talking about giving birth, a narrative form that in large measure eliminates stories of problematic births. She thus hints that, although openness about childbirth is recommended in Swedish society, it also has a regulatory function. The openness about sexuality works in a similar way. The sexual sphere, which is ventilated in such detail particularly in the Swedish mass media, is a subject of public interest which has many points of contact with the control of sexuality that the state and the church zealously exercised for centuries, Bäckman argues.

In Greece it has not been the same ways to control people's private and intimate relations that have dominated. Nor has a public discourse about openness in matters of sexuality and personal relationships been institutionalized to the same extent. Education has not been the goal of any popular movement in Greece as it has in Sweden. Nor has the idea of dialogue about childbirth and parenthood been initiated by Greek authorities. There is no sex education in schools, nor any education about childbirth in parents' groups of the type that is now the rule in Sweden. The sociologist Demosthenes Agrafiotis and his research group at the National School of Public Health in Athens do not single out the Greek Orthodox church or any other institution as having the main responsibility for how sexuality is regulated in the country. Instead they emphasize the significance of the still not totally abandoned agrarian societal order as an important social and cultural context. Surveys show that extramarital relations are now accepted, but that boys often have their first sexual experience in brothels.

In a collection of articles about their own research efforts on HIV/AIDS and sexuality, the authors point out that no systematic studies of sexuality in Greece had yet been conducted by the mid-1990s (Agrafiotis et al., 1997, p. 96). In the same volume we see a picture of sexual habits and attitudes that differ in several respects from the situation in Sweden. This impression is further underlined in my interviews with individual members of the research group at the National School of Public Health in Athens. For instance, the use of contraceptives is rare in lasting relationships, which is explained by the fact that contraceptives are associated by many people with infidelity, and to use them would be regarded as showing lack of trust. Because many people have unsafe sex, abortions are used as a retroactive form of contraception, with the consequence that young women have often had several abortions. (The Greek Gynaecological Association estimates that about 200,000 abortions are performed annually in Greece. The figure is uncertain, however, since the majority of abortions are performed illegally and therefore not registered.)

The authors also point out that homosexuality, until very recently, had seen no research at all in Greece, stating as a reason that Greek society is not yet mature enough to accept homosexuality (Agrafiotis et al., 1997, pp. 152ff). The authors' own quantitative study of sexual habits presented in the same volume simultaneously gives the impression of a sexually active population, but this is not reflected in openness about sexuality. A large proportion of the men who have stated that they have sex with men are married to women and act as heterosexuals, with their own family as a cover (p. 154). As a consequence of this silence, it is not unusual that men who have been infected with HIV by having sex with men prefer to say that they caught the infection by having sex with prostitutes. This situation is confirmed in several interviews, for example, with staff from the AIDS centre in Athens (*Tilefoniki Ghrammi ke Simvoleftikós Stathmós ja to AIDS*). Like Agrafiotis's research group, one can search for structural conditions to explain the relative closedness about sexuality in Greece. Against that background, the silences about HIV can have different expressions and implications in Sweden and Greece. The predominant voice in the Greek public debate does not seem to generate ideas about the value of institutionalizing forms for openness about sensitive personal matters to the same degree as in Sweden.

Two tendencies in the attitudes to suffering have dominated the debate about HIV in Sweden since the end of the 1900s. One is the medicalization of the mental and social consequences of the disease as a consequence of the progress of medical science in curbing HIV/AIDS. Whereas medicine used to be able only to give relief and consolation, effective medical treatment has now sometimes had a tendency to abandon the former "bedside medicine." The other tendency can be described as an increased interest in patients' narratives shown in clinical work. This interest has helped to reveal what happens in the encounter between the voice of medicine and that of the life world (Frank, 1997, pp. 1ff; cf. Charon, 1994, 2006; Kleinman, 1988). Studies have revealed how an asymmetry often arises in conversations between patients and doctors, as a result of which the patients' narratives and interpretations are not given sufficient scope in clinical encounters (Mishler, 1984).

In the transformation that is dissolving the small-scale agrarian community in which Theodora's family originated, older forms of what could be called the culture of suffering clash with newer ones. These cultural changes are expressed in the partly ambivalent attitudes that Theodora's mother showed when she described the family's past and the current powerlessness about being able to support their daughter. The significance of cultural differences for what it is like to be a relative of a person with HIV should therefore not be interpreted on evolutionist premises, but merely as showing that experiences of disease are influenced by a cultural and moral landscape which shapes relations between people's suffering, self-understanding, and moral properties. I shall try to shed light on these relations by comparing Theodora's mother with a Swedish mother of three sons whose eldest son has HIV.

The Swedish woman, whom I call Inger, comes from a rural setting in Sweden, but has lived most of her life in big cities in the United States and later in Greece and Sweden. For periods of varying length she has also lived in other parts of the world, as a consequence of her international assignments. During her second marriage to a Greek-American she lived at times in Greece, where she had a son and a daughter. She divorced for the second time in 1990 and now lives alone in a single-family house in the suburbs of Stockholm. I came into contact with her through our mutual friends in Sweden who have links with Greece. My first interview with Inger had a different framework from that with Panayota. I had known her for a long time and through the years we had become good friends. On one occasion when my study came up in conversation, Inger told me in confidence that her eldest son, Eric, was HIV-positive. I had not met Eric, who lives in the United States, only her daughter and son in Sweden. But since the siblings have not been informed that Eric has HIV, I have not been able to interview them. Inger is therefore the only member of Eric's family whom I have been able to interview. I got to know her as a very spontaneous and outspoken person, and I was surprised to find out how closed she been about Eric's homosexuality among our mutual friends, and the disciplined silence she observed about his HIV infection. She explained that I was the third person in Sweden to find out that Eric has HIV, although 8 years have passed since he received his diagnosis.

Her reasons for keeping silent about Eric's HIV infection were complex and varied according to the situation. One explanation she gave for not having spoken about the subject with her two youngest children was that Eric himself had not wanted them to know. But Inger could not explain why Eric kept silent for them about his infection, whereas he was open about it to many of the people around him in the United States. Nor could she give a simple explanation why she herself had been so silent with family and friends in Sweden about Eric's predicament. The interview instead became a narrative reflecting on how Eric's HIV infection intervened in many contexts of meaning.

The first context she focused on was the divorce from Eric's father, Charles. The divorce had led to a bitter judicial process about who should have custody of Eric, who was then 5 years old. "A relevant factor," Inger told me, "is that Charles is homosexual." It was this insight that had caused the divorce and evidently contributed to her silence, especially among family and friends in Sweden, about Eric's sexuality and his HIV infection. I never understood how these realities were connected, perhaps because Inger omitted important information for me. She made it clear that there were things she was not willing to bring up, events that she would prefer to be forgotten. She also emphasized that Eric's HIV infection, oddly enough, had led to peace between the two people who had been such enemies at the time of the divorce. She also said that Eric's involvement as a volunteer in a soup kitchen providing meals for people with HIV/AIDS had brought him together with his new partner, with whom he is now living happily. She told me how Eric's great sorrow at the start of his HIV infection had been that he did not think he would be able to continue with his demanding job. To his and her great delight, however, the medicines had instead enabled him to enjoy considerable new success in his profession.

In Inger's circle of friends and acquaintances there are few people who know that Eric is living together with a man, let alone that they met at a soup kitchen for people with HIV/AIDS. She has told even fewer people that her first husband was homosexual and that the two contestants in the bitter custody trial have stopped maligning each other as a consequence of Eric's HIV infection. One explanation that Inger gave for having been so silent about Eric's sexuality among her Swedish friends was that she had found the attitude to homosexuality so terribly naïve in Sweden, particularly in feminist circles. She said that she had not found anyone with whom she felt sufficient understanding. She also reflected on what the outlook on homosexuality had done to her generation. She pointed out how she had been confronted with theories which portrayed homosexuality among men as an undesired result of overprotective, frustrated mothers. Inger said that it is not particularly acceptable to be a parent of homosexual children and that HIV, which we have learned to regard as a terrible disease, can seem like a punishment for all the errors that have been committed.

If we test for a moment the idea that both Eric's and Theodora's HIV infections could be regarded as punishments for mistakes, what does this say about the cultural and moral landscape surrounding them and their parents? When it comes to Theodora, the idea would probably be that her infection can be perceived as a punishment for her grandfather's abduction of his bride and the curses that then, according to Panayota's and Aris's narratives, were pronounced on the perpetrator and his family. But rather than the idea of the HIV infection as a punishment uniting the two mothers, we see significant differences. In Eric's case the punishment would be for his mother's personal "errors," making her to blame for his disease. From that point of view her silence about the infection could be interpreted as her way to protect her own and Eric's identity. Panayota's and Aris's narratives single out the abduction as the event that triggered the curses pronounced on their family. If the family through its silence about Theodora's HIV infection wants to avoid any connection between the story of the abduction and the family's current situation, the family members are not primarily protecting their identity as individuals, but rather their collective identity as members of the family.

The picture of differences in their identity formation was also illustrated in a follow-up interview with Inger 6 months later. She made it even more clear that her silences about Eric's sexuality, and in particular his HIV infection, were not caused by external circumstances but by the fact that different realities collided in her own self-understanding. "It's in my head that I can't keep it separated!," she exclaimed when I said that I did not understand what her first divorce, the public mudslinging in the custody dispute, and her first husband's sexuality had to do with her silence about Eric's HIV infection. Panayota, on the other hand, confirmed that openness about Theodora's disease could not be combined with family life. She explained that her husband would not have consented to her participation in an interview about this subject and underlined the importance of keeping the knowledge of her daughter's HIV infection within the family walls in order to protect the whole family from a shameful and painful identity.

Making HIV into a family secret in this way puts the spotlight on what can be perceived as the family's most intimate core: the physical, social, and cultural reproduction of its members. On a general level, family secrets can thereby be regarded as the other side of the family's outward face (Davidoff et al., 1999, p. 244). But being silent as Inger was about Eric's HIV infection because, as she said, she wanted to protect herself against lack of understanding about homosexuality, particularly in some feminist circles, concerns another kind of identity problem. Her silence was also about relating to circles outside her family, but in this context the problem concerns how she is valued and how she values herself as a woman and mother, rather than how her family is valued. Based on these comparisons, one cannot draw firm conclusions about Inger's and Panayota's actual experiences of having a family member with HIV.

An impression that stayed with me, however, is that they were both critical or ambivalent to dominant ideas about the relationship between openness, closedness, and suffering in their cultural surroundings. In Panayota's narrative about family life she was critical that they had accepted an order which did not give any scope for intimate relations between the members of the family. In Inger's narrative about her family, she made it clear that she wished certain things to be forgotten. At the same time, she herself seemed somewhat surprised that she surrounded Eric's sexuality and HIV infection with so much silence in her life in Sweden. She was not especially anxious, as Panayota was, to extend her opportunities to speak about personal matters. In this respect their different narratives indicate the significance of cultural differences in their total life situations. The most striking thing is that, unlike Panayota, Inger has left her rural beginnings and moved between different cultural contexts in different cities. In that sense Inger was more accustomed to moving between many very different realities. She was therefore probably more familiar with separating the different worlds of which she was part, without this having to be done at the expense of scope for intimacy. Nevertheless the way people follow or negotiate cultural agreements concerning what could be told openly or ought to be kept silent about, reflect cultural differences. Exploring silences in terms of broken narratives, therefore, can be a way of interpreting cultural differenses.

CONCLUDING REMARKS

The fact that narratives are broken stands out in my study as a consequence of the fact that they often give rise to conflicts and social dynamics. The statement that narratives and silences shape the conditions for what it is like to live with HIV/AIDS proceeds from well-documented observations in several spheres that narratives an d silences are both locally and globally distributed and active on many levels. Even if individuals with HIV/AIDS and their relatives have different attitudes to speaking openly or keeping the disease secret, no one can remain unaffected by the silence that surrounds the disease in many contexts around the world. I have given examples of how narratives tie different realities together, while silences separate them from each other. In the Greek family to which I have referred, I have pointed out conceivable unwelcome associations between the story of Theodora's HIV diagnosis and the almost mythological tale of how her grandfather abducted his bride. This also concerns in large measure the link between her HIV diagnosis and the narrative of her relationship with Petros, his past, and his death from AIDS. The different attitudes of the family members to this relationship show that both narratives and demands for silence can engender conflicts and give rise to social dynamics. The breach of confidentiality concerning Theodora's diagnosis illustrates, moreover, how an unwelcome narrative can break forth and change the conditions for living with the disease and being a next of kin.

As an analytical concept, broken narratives offer a possibility to problematize the relationship between narratives and silences and make silences empirically analysable. Raising questions about broken narratives can give insight into the communicative contexts surrounding the narration. These contexts, as I have said, include narratives which can have undesired consequences if they are linked to each other. Examining that type of link can make silences comprehensible. The study of broken narratives can thereby be a way to problematize people's evasive strategies and the relationship between their narratives and silences. One justification for this statement is that I have given the concept of broken narratives a broad meaning, based on the understanding of narratives as constituting reality. If all narratives contain a broken narrative in some sense, they can also draw attention to the absent voices and to the interaction between narratives and silences at different levels.

As a perspective, broken narratives speak to an action-oriented understanding of narratives and silences. I have tried to show this by describing broken narratives as embodied everyday cultural practices. As such, silences are like narratives in being the result of the conscious actions of different actors. Broken narratives, like "unbroken" ones, do something. My example has shown that broken narratives can both cause and prevent suffering. Countless testimonies all over the world also show clearly that the suffering which the disease can cause should not only be regarded as a problem on an individual level. An excessively narrow field of vision obscures the picture of how the social suffering that can accompany the situation of next of kin is influenced by political, economic, institutional, and other forces surrounding the disease (cf. Kleinman, Das & Lock, 1997, p. ix). Expanding the meaning of broken narratives in connection with HIV/AIDS can therefore also be justified by a will to understand how the conditions for living with the disease are affected by these broader contexts.

ACKNOWLEDGMENTS

The research project was carried out with support from the Bank of Sweden Tercentenary Foundation. I would like to thank Professor Barbro Klein, The Swedish Collegium for Advanced Study (SCAS), for helpful reading of an earlier version of this chapter.

A NOTE ON TRANSCRIPTION CONVENTIONS

In the transcribed extracts from the interview I have used the following conventions:

Interrupted utterance: a slash after the utterance/

An incomplete utterance ends with two dots. .

Drawn-out words: a dash after the word—

Interjected acknowledgement, objections: [in brackets]

Interjected questions, or start of questions: [¿question]

My comments: (in parentheses)

Words or phrases in later quotations which are quoted in Greek are transcribed according to phonetic principles and rendered in Latin letters. Some of the ability of the transcription to convey the oral style gets lost in translation, especially in the later quotations of Alkisti's speech and narrative, which were first translated by me into Swedish and later rendered in English by a professional translator. The analysis, however, is based on my listening to the recorded interviews and reading the transcriptions in Greek and Swedish.

REFERENCES

Agrafiotis, D. et al. (1997). Aids. Engársia skiá: koinonikó-polistikés kai psycholoyikés diastaséis. Aten: Ýpsilon Vivlía.

Bäckman, M. (2003). *Kön och känsla: Samlevnadsundervisning och ungdomars tankar om sexualitet.* Stockholm: Makadam Förlag.

Bendix, R. (2003). Sleepers' secrets, actors' revelations. *Ethnologia Europaea, 33,* 33–42.

Briggs, C., & Mantini-Briggs, C. (2003). *Stories in the time of cholera: Racial profiling during a medical nightmare.* Berkeley, CA: University of California Press.

Campbell, J. (1976). *Honour, family, and patronage: A study of institutions and moral values in a Greek mountain community.* New York: Oxford University Press.

Charon, R. (1994). Narrative contributions to medical ethics: Recognition, formulation, interpretation, and validation in the practice of the ethicist. In E. R. DuBose, R. P. Hamel, & L. J. O'Connel (Eds.), *A matter of principles? Ferment in U.S. bioethics* (pp. 260–83). Valley Forge, PA: Trinity Press International.

Charon, R. (2006). *Narrative medicine: Honoring the stories of illness.* New York: Oxford University Press.

Davidoff, L., et al. (1999). *The family story: Blood, contract and intimacy 1830– 1960.* London: Longman.

Drakos, G. (1997). *Makt över kropp och hälsa: Om leprasjukas självförståelse i dagens Grekland.* Stockholm/Stehag: Östlings bokförlag Symposion.

Drakos, G. (2005). Berättelsen i sjukdomens värld: Att leva med hiv/aids som anhörig i Sverige och Grekland. Stockholm/Stehag: Östlings bokförlag Symposion.

Drakos, G. (2006). HIV/AIDS, narrativity and embodiment. In A. Kaivola-Bregenhøj, B. Klein, & U. Palmenfelt (Eds.), *Narrating, doing, experiencing. Nordic folkloristic perspectives.* Helsinki, Finland: Studia Fennica Folkloristica.

Frank, A. W. (1997). *The wounded storyteller: Body, illness, and ethics.* Chicago: The University of Chicago Press.

Friedl, E. (1962). *Vasilika: A village in modern Greece.* New York: Holt, Rinehart, and Winston.

Friedl, E. (1986). The position of women: Appearance and reality. In J. Dubisch (Ed.), *Gender and power in rural Greece.* Princeton, NJ: Princeton University Press.

Goffman, E. (1959). *The presentation of self in everyday life.* New York: Doubleday.

Herzfeld, M. (1988). *The poetics of manhood: Contest and identity in a Cretan mountain village.* Princeton, NJ: Princeton University Press.

Herzfeld, M. (1991). Silence, submission, and subversion: Toward a poetics of womanhood. In P. Loizos & E. Papataxiarchis (Eds.), *Contested identities: Gender and kinship in modern Greece.* Princeton, NJ: Princeton University Press.

Kirmayer, L. J. (2000). Broken narratives: Clinical encounters and the poetics of illness experience. In C. Mattingly & L. C. Garro (Eds.), *Narrative and the cultural construction of illness and healing.* Berkeley, CA: University of California Press.

Kleinman, A. (1988). *The illness narratives: Suffering, healing and the human condition.* New York: Basic Books.

Kleinman, A., Das, V., & Lock, M. (1997). *Social suffering.* Berkeley, CA: University of California Press.

Mishler, E. G. (1984). *The discourse of medicine: Dialectics of medical interviews.* Norwood, NJ: Ablex.

Nylund Skog, S. (2002). Ambivalenta upplevelser & mångtydiga berättelser: En etnologisk studie av barnafödande. Stockholms Universitet: Etnologiska institutionen.

Seremetakis, C. N. (1991). *The last word: Women, death, and divination in inner Mani.* Chicago: The University of Chicago Press.

Simmel, G. (1999). Das Geheimnis und die geheime Gesellschaft. In *Soziologie: Untersuchungen über Formen der Vergesellschaftung. Simmel Gesamtausgaube,* (Vol. 2, pp. 383–455). Frankfurt, Germany: Suhkamp.

Stylianoudi, M-G. L. (1996). Genogram as narrative: Interpreting genograms, *European Journal for Semiotic Studies, 8,* 775–793.

7   Caring for the Dead
Broken Narratives of Internment

Arthur W. Frank

Stories enact grief. Stories not only describe the storyteller's life after a loved one has died; they are, in their telling, *acts* of grieving. By telling others what has happened, the storyteller as *witness* to suffering tells himself or herself. As storytellers hear themselves tell their stories, they become able to know their own experiences in a new way. They establish an attitude toward an event that *becomes* the experience of that event. *Experience* comes to be through the storytelling process. Grief is an experience, and so is healing. Whatever this overused, near-cliché word *healing* may mean, it seems to involve capacity of stories to shift experience—the event always changing in repeated acts of storytelling.

The sort of *broken narratives* that I am most concerned with are stories that resist telling; stories that the storyteller resists hearing himself or herself tell. The storyteller may self-consciously reflect on that resistance and make those reflections part of the story, or the storytelling may display resistance in gaps, inconsistencies, and other overt breaks in the narrative flow. In a broken narrative, emotions *fracture* the telling, and the listener or reader is left with fragments that do not form a whole, or the whole they form has holes in it. The narratives that concern me are broken because *the nature of the experience does not, cannot, and never will coalesce into a cohesive whole,* as narrative traditions expect wholeness. The storyteller struggles between a need to let the story act as a form of what grief counselors would call *closure,* and opposed to that, a sense that any story presenting the experience as complete and completed would betray what happened and betray what the imperative of witness demands.

The concept of broken narratives directs our attention to a story's *liminality;* an anthropological term referring to physical spaces outside the safe boundaries of a village enclosure and to rituals in which participants are between fixed roles (Turner, 1969). Liminal spaces are *neither here nor there,* and they are *dangerous.* Narratives become broken not when they are *about* such spaces, but rather when the narrative is told from *within* liminal spaces. Such narratives call upon the reader or listener to enter their space. Reading or hearing a broken narrative, we, as readers or listeners, feel pulled across some boundary that we did not want to cross, into a zone where life is profoundly insecure. Yet the story holds us, making it safe enough—not entirely safe but compelling—to follow where it leads.

A further aspect of the story's brokenness lies in the *relationship* between storyteller and listener. Unbroken narratives develop a complicity of mutual understanding. As these stories are told, the initial gap or distance between storyteller and listeners diminishes; each feels increasingly secure in the knowledge of the other. In broken narratives, the listeners realize that they remain on the edges of an experience they can never comprehend. *You are on one side,* the story reminds us, *and this other human being is on another side. Whatever you hear in this story, or think you hear, a gap will remain between your experience and what is being told. The brokenness is your inability to close that gap, either by believing that now you know what the storyteller lived through and thus claiming that experience as part of wholeness of your life, or by going back to life as you lived it before you heard the story.*

*

The broken narratives that I want to discuss are both by fathers whose newborn sons have died. William Kotzwinkle published an early version of *Swimmer in a Silent Sea* as a magazine short story in the early 1970s, and it appeared as a novella in 1994. *Swimmer in a Silent Sea* is written in the third person and presented as a work of fiction. I find myself reluctant to seek to find out how much of the story is autobiographical. Investigative research, at least in this instance, seems to undermine the author's choice of genre, because it expresses a commitment to the author's personal involvement in the story's events. Once that assumption is made, it can never be entirely disproven. If the author had wanted to identify himself as the protagonist, he would have. The other story is by George Michelson Foy, also a novelist, who does write in the first person. Foy's nonfiction story, "Burning Olivier," was published in *Harper's* magazine in 1999. The two stories are strikingly similar in how each protagonist—the character Laski in Kotzwinkle's novella and Foy in his story—reacts to the death of his son.

The son in Kotzwinkle's story, who is never named, dies at birth in a small hospital in rural Maine. There is no apparent reason for this death; the baby simply never breathes. The birth is a breach delivery, but that is handled with skill. Even after an autopsy, all the physicians can say is that it was bad luck. Foy's son, Olivier, lives for a month in the Neonatal Intensive Care Unit at Children's Hospital in Boston. Olivier appears normal at birth, but after his first day, heart problems become apparent that quickly make his life dependent on complex NICU machinery. Finally, Foy makes a decision to turn off life-support, and Olivier dies in his arms.

Each man then makes a fateful decision to bury his son himself. "I see it as anathema," Foy (1999) writes, using a word with provocative theological connotations, "that the final send-off of people whose stories you care about should be placed in the hands of those who must manufacture the emotions that connect them to the dead" (p. 40). Foy is devastating in his objections to professional funeral homes, which he understands as financially exploitative. "These 'homes,'" he writes, putting *homes* in scare quotes, "are utterly devoid of the type of individual and affectionate care that Olivier enjoyed throughout his abbreviated life. There was no way in hell I was going to let the cold hands of those franchised carrion-feeders come anywhere near my son" (p. 41). Strong words, perhaps necessary to summon the resolve required for such a weighty decision.

Kotzwinkle's hero Laski is less political in his objections to funeral homes. He contemplates having a funeral home cremate his son, but when he is driving up to it, a funeral is taking place. Laski sees what he describes as "a crew of professionally somber men in black." He drives past the home, "horrified," asking himself, "What in hell did I almost do?" (pp. 70–71). Later he explains the funeral home idea to his wife as, "Just something I dreamed up to protect myself from the truth of death" (p. 72). Foy and Laski both choose to confront the truth of death—whatever that may be—without this protection of conventional, and commercialized, practice. Both narratives are animated by the reader's fear and hope for how the protagonist's decision will turn out: Will such a step precipitate disaster or healing? In any narrative, one thing leads to another, and the story teaches what sort of things lead to what other sort of things. In broken narratives, the chaining of acts is complex. One act has multiple consequences, and the moral valence of those consequences is not immediately clear. Good and bad happens together, and normal moral or therapeutic terms of evaluation are called into question. As actions take place in Foy's and Kotzwinkle's stories, necessity trumps desirability; both stories neither recommend nor caution against their response to death. Each reports only what *had* to be.

How Laski and Foy act depends on both the conditions of their respective son's deaths and the legal-bureaucratic situation each finds himself in. Laski's son is born almost already dead but not quite. As Laski drives home from the hospital, "he felt the spirit of his son spreading out all around him. Spreading out as it did, into every tree and cloud, he felt it losing personality, felt it dissolving into something remote, expanding beyond his powers to follow. He's going now, thought Laski" (p. 52). Laski finds himself in this space in which his son is dead but not yet departed, because it has all happened too fast. Too many boundaries have been crossed too quickly; the crossings are incomplete. Part of Laski's son is on one side, and part on the other, and Laski is with him on both sides. Laski's son has always existed more in his imagination, as a potential. Laski has not spent every day for a month, as Foy has, holding an actual child, talking to that child, imagining what the child is experiencing, and finally making a decision that this experience is not life, so there must be death.

In death, care must continue. When Olivier has died, the nurse begins to fold him into a blanket. Foy stops her, and she understands immediately that he wants to do it. "It felt good to me that I could take care of my boy's body even after he had stopped breathing," Foy writes (p. 42). He holds Olivier for several minutes, and then asks the nurse where he should put the body, expecting her to wheel it away on a gurney. Instead, in an extraordinary act of care, the nurse takes the baby in her arms. "And she put him to her shoulder the way a mother would burp her child, one hand supporting his back and neck. 'He's still just a baby,' she said" (p. 42).

As a culmination to this slow, deliberate process of caring, death is momentous but not so clear a boundary as might have been imagined or feared, and Foy no less than Laski finds himself within a space between life and death. The problem Foy sets for himself is how to continue to give Olivier the same level of care that the nurse exhibits, throughout what he calls his son's "final send-off." Continuing to care for Olivier is a form of care for himself; he writes, "one could not abandon a child at any stage without jumping ship on part of oneself" (p. 41). When he encounters bureaucratic obstacles that others would find formidable, he experiences them as vaguely therapeutic. "Perhaps the most useful aspect of the do-it-yourself funeral approach," Foy writes, "was that it dragged me backward into the process to the world where I had spent the last month—the cosmos of hospitals, of Boston, of medical rules and personnel—of which Olivier, alive or dead, remained the astronomical pole" (p. 46). In the sameness of procedure, Olivier remains the guiding presence.

Laski is able to cut through various bureaucratic procedures more quickly, in part because of the rapidity of his son's death, and in part because he is in rural Maine. Laski, for whom events have moved more quickly, acts without Foy's degree of reflection about what compels him. He rejects the intrusion of self-reflection with a Zen-like appeal to being entirely in the present action. Once at home, he begins building a casket for his son: "I built a house for us, with a room for him, and now I'm building his casket. There's no difference in the work. We simply must go along, eyes open, watching our work carefully, *without any extra thoughts*" (p. 66, emphases added).

A focal scene in both stories is each man building a box in which his son will be placed; that building is a physical work that each man finds beneficial. Laski sees "that it was a good thing to do, that it was a privilege few men had anymore. He marked the line carefully and sawed a matching piece to form the floor of the casket" (p. 66). "I do it quietly," Laski says to himself, "not even for him, for he's gone beyond my little box. But he left behind a fragment of himself, which requires a box that I can carry through the woods. And a box needs a lid and I've got to find a pair of hinges" (p. 67). Laski's clarity of focus on the task at hand reminds me of the Zen story of the student who asked the Master about enlightenment. "Have you had dinner?" the Master asked in reply. When the student said he had, the Master told him, "Wash you bowl," that counting as an answer to the original question about enlightenment. A box needs a lid, and the lid needs hinges; those are sufficient to occupy a person, without any "extra thoughts."

Foy, who lacks at least Laski's carpentry tools, enlists a friend to help him build the box in which Olivier will be cremated, because for Foy and his wife to be able to bury their son themselves, cremation at a funeral home is legally required, hence the title, "Burning Olivier." If the nurse who carries Olivier on her shoulder is one moral guide in Foy's story, another guide is the friend, Peter, who helps build the casket. The complement to the nurse's moral reminder, "He's still just a baby," is Peter correcting Foy's initial choice of which wood is appropriate for the task. "You can't use *plywood*," Peter says, to which Foy adds, "What he means is, You don't use mass-produced industrial shortcuts—alternatives to milled planks and the painstaking attention of hands—for work that means a great deal to you" (p. 50).

Foy, possibly because of the month he has spent with Olivier and possibly because of who he is, is haunted by the "extra thoughts" of what will happen once Olivier is buried. Then he will confront what he calls "the beast." "And the beast is, quite simply, missing him, knowing he will not be with you ever again except in the makeshift and unworthy stories you tell" (p. 51). We, Foy's readers, are of course reading one of those stories, and the story becomes a metaphorical extension of the box. Foy's observation that "the tactile joy that comes from building [the box] is something that Olivier's death cannot entirely subtract from me" (p. 50), carries forward in time to his later act of writing, which is a tactile joy of seeing words appear.

The idea that words, writing, and storytelling can offer a kind of solace to death brings me to the most perilous theme in any discussion of bereavement, which is what is often called *recovery*. The brokenness of Kotzwinkle's and Foy's narratives lies in their disruption of both the expected trajectory and the means of recovery. What is broken is the conventional promise—whether psychological or theological—that people *can* recover from such losses. To understand this brokenness, we need to consider how stories depend on and reassert that conventional promise; specifically, we need a template for an *unbroken* narrative of death and bereavement.

*

The unbroken narrative is described on the jacket of Kotzwinkle's book by a publicist who knows pretty well what the reading public expects from a narrative about death, and his or her blurb is one of the multitude of small gestures the cumulative force of which recreates that expectation. Kotzwinkle's book, the blurb says, "portrays one family's loss, acceptance, and, ultimately, affirmation." This utterly conventional description depends on the default assumption that bereavement is supposed to proceed through generic stages of loss, acceptance, and ultimate affirmation. Whether or not Elizabeth Kübler-Ross (1969) was an adequate observer of dying, or an adequate therapist to the dying, she has unquestionably been, for the last half century, the great narrator of dying, at least in Western countries.

Perhaps she might more accurately be called a *narrativist*, not a narrator who tells specific stories, but someone whose work has the force of setting a template for how stories are to be told. In this template, loss is progressively transformed into restored wholeness, whether this restoration is called closure, recovery, or acceptance. Transformation is imagined as a progression, which is made manageable by taking place in observable, discrete stages.

The unbroken narrative imagines an original wholeness, the loss of that wholeness, and some actions that constitute a metaphorical or real journey in response to that loss. At the end of this journey is a renewed wholeness that is *sadder but wiser,* in the famous closing words of S. T. Coleridge's great poem of suffering and storytelling, "The Rime of the Ancient Mariner." Coleridge is another of our great narrativists of suffering, whose story has become a template for future storytelling. Of course Coleridge did not invent the template, any more than Kübler-Ross discovered anything that was new. She transformed the poetic story into a list that anticipates the Power Point slide and, again, renders the process *more manageable* by showing people where they are, on the way to a promised resolution.

The loss and regaining of wholeness is probably humanity's oldest story. The mythologist Joseph Campbell (1973) describes the hero's journey in stages that are readily evident in both Foy's and Kotzwinkle's narratives. The hero first hears a *call,* which she or he initially resists but then is forced to acknowledge. Responding to the call requires a *descent* with a sequence of *trials* through which the hero must persevere; Campbell's most ancient mythological heroes do not triumph so much as they *persevere* through suffering. The hero typically finds a *helper,* who at first seems an unlikely ally but eventually helps the hero to *return,* which is penultimate to receiving what Campbell calls the *boon,* a reward that is often more spiritual than material—in the post-Romantic age of individualism, the boon is a personal *transformation* that results from suffering. The hero attempts to make this boon available to those to whom she or he has returned, and the sad but wise closing of the story is other people's refusal of what could save them, or more exactly, their inability to perceive the value of what is being offered. Transformation requires making the journey *oneself.*

Foy's and Kotzwinkle's stories follow Campbell's narrative trajectory in some respects, but both narratives break with the journey of suffering leading to the boon of transformation, and herein lies both narratives' brokenness. As Laski's wife is nearing the end of her labor, he imagines that he and she are on the edge of a Campbell-like return: "He felt them together, then, on a new level, older, wiser, with pain as the binder in their union" (pp. 16–17). This is the "acceptance" that the publisher's blurb promises, but it occurs on page 16 of a 90-page novella. Close to the story's end, the certainty of time and trajectory that are implicit in the idea of the couple *moving,* through the pain of labor, to a "new level" is gone, utterly deflated by what has happened. "Laski lowered the lid of the box, and again it seemed like a dream that could move in any direction he willed. But then he felt reality moving in only one direction. The baby was born and he died and I'm closing the lid of his coffin" (p. 85). Time moves not as Laski will, and the events do not lead to some *telos* of insight. Any boon is as dark as it is light.

Foy's story is more explicitly broken. He turns Campbell's journey into an interactive process of one level of descent precipitating a further descent, with points of interruption between spirals. The suspense of the story is how long any of these interruptions will last, and how far down the descent will go. Foy's fear is that literally closing the lid on Olivier will be the moment when his descent will become an uncontrolled free fall. At that moment he will lack what sustains and perhaps restrains him at present, which are material possibilities for continuing to care for Olivier. Here are Foy's "extra thoughts" that Laski works to exclude, but that may affect him as well.

> Along with [the fear of never physically being able to touch or see my boy again] rose another flavor of fear, because it was almost ten days now since Olivier had died. In that time I had sprinted headlong down the path I had chosen, of taking care of Olivier—knowing, yet ignoring the knowledge, that when the process was finally ended, when my son was finally burned, the unexcised shadow of missing him must fold me in its immense, bat-like wings and take me down much harder than if I'd never started down the trail. And I was less sure than I had been before if I could survive such an embrace intact. (p. 54)

In Campbell's hero's journey, the return is certain; the genre requires it. The broken narrative resembles a horror film in which the evil force is never fully destroyed, and any provisionally happy ending is experienced in anticipation of that evil's return—until the moviegoer leaves the theater and has the pleasure of relegating the story to the realm of cinematic genre fantasy. The broken narrative offers no such exit into the light of wholeness; the trials will not end, leaving the protagonist to return to life at a new level of wisdom and unity. Moreover, this brokenness, the narrative shows us, is the essence of life.

Foy's return, insofar as it is a return, seems to be made possible as much by storytelling as by the actions of Olivier's cremation and burial. At the end of his story, Foy is visiting a friend who asks him if he will write about Olivier's life and death. Thinking about that, Foy offers what is probably his most explicit gesture in the direction of the conventional unbroken narrative of affirmation: "I also recalled the thought I'd had the morning after he died—that Olivier had given me, and also Liz, the most fully realized living we had ever done—as dense in hope and yearning as it was soaked in fear and pain" (p. 54). This recognition leads to writing: "In some manner, I thought, the greater harm would lie not in forgetting but in not continuing the process" (p. 54). That continuation at least includes the story that the reader is finishing.

Broken narratives intensify the reader's interpretive involvement; at the story's end, the reader has a choice between wholeness and brokenness. Reading the story as one of wholeness understands that Foy's writing finally frees him from the "bat-like wings" that threatened him. Or, if not that, at least writing one story could lead to another, and Foy had found a secure means to sustain himself, a method of narrative self-therapy. The reader who is left wondering, or doubting, whether Foy will be able to "continue the process" beyond the present story understands the narrative as fully broken. In the brokenness reading, any expressions of gratitude, acceptance, and completeness stand as transitory hopes borrowed from stories that Foy can gesture toward but never make his own; the bat-like wings seem more real.

*

The bat wings are made more real by Foy's deprecation of what he calls the "fantasy of fixing" (p. 50). In broken narratives, fixing remains a fantasy. As much as Foy enjoys building the box, and by extension crafting his story, it is too much of a reach to claim any transformation results from either work. Olivier may have given Foy and his wife "the most fully realized living we had ever done" (p. 54), but that claim risks becoming part of a fantasy that something like death can be fixed: "I realize," Foy reflects on building the box, "I am still working off the adolescent fantasy that I can always nail together some cool box, some Rube Goldberg gizmo that will do the trick" (p. 50). Foy's self-recognition returns me to Laski's line about the need to protect ourselves from the truth of death. Truth seems to begin in the recognition that *fixing* often is an adolescent fantasy.

Yet, Foy and Kotzwinkle both end their stories with pastoral descriptions in which the brokenness does seem mitigated. Foy: "Then we buried our son under a young cypress, in the midst of blue myrtle and dogwood and white pine, within sight of Nantucket Sound" (p. 54). Kotzwinkle: "On the slope behind the old barn, the toboggan [on which Laski is carrying his son through the forest to where they will bury him] moved on its own and he ran alongside it, guiding it with the rope through a stand of young spruce. The arms of the little trees touched the box, shedding some needles upon it, and a few tiny cones" (p. 91). Such language makes the narrative whole and repairs the brokenness. But is this repair the "truth of death" from which Laski realizes that funeral homes protect us (p. 72)?

Laski's decision to bury their son has its climactic moment when he and his wife unwrap the boy's body, to look at him one more time before burying him. They have consented to an autopsy, believing that the body would be sewn back together afterwards. When they unfold the linen shroud in which the hospital wrapped the boy's body, they find dirty rags around a garbage bag. Inside, the baby's body remains cut open, the spine visible through the chest cavity. Against my expectations, the child's parents do not seem indignant at how the hospital has treated their son's body; instead, the surgical opening seems to enable a clearer vision of exactly what is. "A fire raged through Laski's body, swelling his chest with blood and burning his throat. 'This is death!' he cried, tears bursting from his eyes. 'There's nothing strange about it!'" (pp. 82–83). "I could look at him forever," says Diane, Laski's wife, the unnamed child's mother (p. 85).

Death is a cold, motionless body, animated by whatever makes a parent want to look forever at the physically broken corpse of her son. The brokenness of these narratives is that beyond their pastoral descriptions of taking the bodies of the dead to what Foy calls their "final send-off" lies the recognition, which is more explicit in Foy's story, that there will be nothing final—no closure—for those who remain behind. Hope for life after lies in this: If the physical reality of death can be gazed upon clearly, there is nothing strange. It is the words, the extra thoughts, that risk confusing us. Laski and Diane are able to tolerate the condition in which the hospital has left their son's body because they see *him*, as he is, without extraneous judgments.

Narratives that show suffering leading to transformation and enriched wholeness use words to point to something ostensibly beyond themselves. The comfort of words lies in that capacity to point beyond, but taking us outside the present moment is also the hollowness of words. Words take us *beyond* the moment of the flesh and its sorrows in both senses: as *transcendence* and as being *beside the point* of what's happening.

In broken narratives, words seem most like the boxes these men build, something one crafts to hold what Kotzwinkle calls fragments that have been left behind (see p. 67). Storytelling, as a way to continue the process of caring, may be the best that anyone can do. The broken narrative is a haunting reminder of what Laski says to Diane while they discuss options for burying their son: "Maybe there isn't any best" (p. 70).

REFERENCES

Campbell, J. (1973). *The hero with a thousand faces*. Princeton, NJ: Princeton University Press. (Original work published 1949)

Foy, G. M. (1999, July). Burning Olivier: The brief life and private burial of an infant son. *Harpers*, 39–54.

Kotzwinkle, W. (1994). *Swimmer in the secret sea*. San Francisco: Chronicle Books.

Kubler-Ross, E. (1969). *On death and dying*. New York: Simon & Schuster.

Turner, V. (1969). *The ritual process: Structure and anti-structure*. Ithaca, NY: Cornell University Press.

8 "You Have to Ask a Little"
Troublesome Storytelling About Contested Illness

Pia Bülow

INTRODUCTION

"Whether ill people want to tell stories or not, illness calls for stories," writes Frank (1995). This need to tell stories when becoming seriously ill is both literal and existential. Literal, since becoming ill in the first place usually means that one has to tell family, doctors, employers, and friends about the way one is feeling bad and how the illness started. The need is existential by the way narratives are used to reconstruct the life story wrecked by serious or chronic illness. Narrating one's illness is thus an act of meaning making. It is something we do to understand and to explain illness—to ourselves as well as to other people. Sometimes, however, telling others about one's suffering might become troublesome.

Some kinds of illnesses about which storytelling might become both problematic and crucial are *contested illnesses* like chronic fatigue syndrome (CFS), fibromyalgia and multiple chemical sensitivity (MCS). Such illnesses are debated and disputed due to insufficient medical explanations and because they are "invisible" and nonobjective, impossible to confirm by traditional medical procedures. Therefore, stories are the most important (perhaps the only) possibility for the ill to claim illness. In the medical encounter, as well as in everyday conversations, illness has to be "storied" to "exist." The story and in what way it is heard could be the difference between receiving a certain diagnosis or not, or between becoming confirmed or doubted. Unless one tells a convincing story, illness becomes contested.

At the same time, telling someone about a condition that is contested means taking a risk. If the sufferer does not succeed in establishing credibility for the story not only illness might become doubted, the person's moral conduct can be called into question. But if what a person tells is not heard as a story about illness—or not even as a story—what happens then to the narration of that storyteller? Can being contested change the way illness is told about or affect an ill person's readiness to narrativize his or her suffering?

During a study about CFS, I conducted a series of interviews with 14 sufferers. These interviews include lots of stories about becoming ill, seeing doctors, feeling doubted, coping with illness, and why the interviewees got ill (for an analysis of these stories see Bülow, 2008). Many of these stories were elaborated and told with what seemed to be great ease. However, for 2 of the men in my study group, the invitation to narrativize illness became troublesome in different ways. One man told elaborated stories about life before and with CFS but could not locate illness in the story of life in the sense that he could not find any kind of explanation for becoming ill. For the other person, a man in his early 30s, the whole series of interviews appeared to me as told in a *broken manner*. On the one hand, I experienced these interviews as rather complicated and demanding, containing few stories about his life. On the other hand, when thinking about these meetings, I felt that I had learned a lot about this man's experiences of illness. This induced me to take a closer look at these interviews. The first man was diagnosed with CFS while the second one did not receive the diagnosis. I asked myself if the difficulties in telling stories about illness were connected to the rejection of diagnosis, or if the troublesome storytelling I experienced merely was a consequence of the interview situation and thus basically a methodological problem, or was it something else that made them appear as broken to me?

In this chapter I discuss difficulties in telling stories about a contested illness like CFS in research interviews but also in medical encounters and in everyday life as was described in the interviews. As an example I use the series of interviews conducted with the second man whom I call Tony. I start with a brief presentation of CFS, describing what it is that makes this a contested illness and move on to illness narratives in general and troublesome storytelling about CFS in particular.

CFS A CONTESTED ILLNESS

CFS is a quite new diagnosis, named and defined in the United States in 1988 (Holmes et al., 1988). It is (together with MCS) described as an emergent illness in the sense that it is "researched, discussed and reported on, but no aspect of [it] is settled medically, legally, or popularly" (Dumit, 2006, p. 578). Even if CFS was defined quite recently, chronic fatigue as a phenomenon has a longer history and CFS has been compared with conditions like neurasthenia (cf. Rabinbach, 1992; Ware & Kleinman, 1992). Just like neurasthenia, CFS is commonly described as an illness mostly affecting women: About 70% are women and 30% men among those diagnosed with CFS (Evengård, Schacterle, & Komaroff, 1999). People do not die of CFS and it is not an illness involving progressive deterioration. Still it is connected with rather poor prognosis—about 10% return to the same functional level as before illness (Joyce, Hotopf, & Wessely, 1997). Most sufferers are ill for a very long time and the condition profoundly affects their life since most them are unable to work in the same way as they used to do.

The main reason for CFS being a contested illness is probably that diagnosis is received from subjective symptoms, which the patient reports. Aside from a medically unexplained fatigue that is persistent or relapsing for at least 6 months, four or more of the following symptoms should be part of that report: headache, sore throat, painful lymph glands, muscle pain, joint pain, unrefreshing sleep, postexertion malaise, and cognitive problems severe enough to cause a considerable decrease in activity (Fukuda et al., 1994). None of these symptoms is possible to check through objective medical tests. Instead, CFS is a diagnosis of exclusion. Clinicians cannot prove that a person *has* CFS. They can only rule out other disorders that the patient does *not have*. In the end, the diagnosis is reached through interactive processes largely based on the story of illness presented by the patient and interpreted by the physician (Hydén & Sachs, 1998).

TELLING STORIES ABOUT ILLNESS

Illness narratives are stories dealing with the experience of illness told by sufferers, by their kin, or by professionals working with patients like physicians, nurses, and occupational therapists (Hydén, 1997; Hydén & Bülow, 2006). Such narratives may include any kind of experience due to illness like issues about when and why someone has become ill, what illness means, the reaction of other people, and how to deal with illness. Furthermore, illness narratives explain, account for, and make sense of illness and actions toward illness. They include questions about identity, moral issues like responsibility, and changed perspectives (cf. Bülow, 2008; Bülow & Hydén, 2003a). Such narratives can be found in encounters at clinics, in books, on the Internet, and in research interviews.

In order to study narratives about illness by interviewing, we might assume, just as Linde (1993) who argues for life stories in general, that most ill people "have" a narrative to tell and that such stories are something people create to make sense of life, to draw new maps for their lives and to connect their past with what is happening due to the illness–thus making the life story coherent. As researchers, this might give us the idea that we just have to evoke these stories. But is it really that simple?

Troublesome storytelling

Besides the interviews, my study about CFS comprised an observation study of a group activity for patients arranged by a clinic specialized in CFS—a so-called *patient school* (Bülow, 2004; Bülow & Hydén, 2003b). This "school" for people suffering from CFS or similar illnesses included lectures about CFS held by medical professionals and group talk guided by a nurse. The interviewees, 10 women and 4 men, were all former participants in the patient school. This means that I had met all of the interviewees already before the first interview with each of them. They were all, with one exception, interviewed twice or on three occasions.

In all three interviews with Tony, I had the impression that it was difficult for him to tell me about his illness. Not that he refused to answer my questions or declined to respond to my invitation to narrate. Neither did he seem to hesitate about participating in the study in the first place. On the contrary, he seemed anxious to contribute with his experiences. His willingness to do so was shown at the end of the first interview when I, after about 40 minutes of interviewing and partly because of my impression that the situation was a bit complicated, asked him if we should turn off the recorder. "No, ask me more. Take this chance," he answered and added, when I hypothetically suggested that sometimes one could feel that now it is enough. "No, I can tell you everything, it's not really that (.) You can ask me anything." Except this eagerness, the story he was telling me about suffering from CFS seemed to be told in a broken manner. By this I mean that it was told in a tentative and tottering way. This was most evident in the first interview but my impression remained during the second and third interview. It was as if he was not used to formulating his personal experiences of illness into a story. Maybe this was what he meant by "*it's not really that*" at the end of the first interview.

The problem of beginning a story

A particular problem when narrating one's chronic illness concerns the fact that one is still in the middle of the story, as Good and Good argue (1994). When asked to tell a story of one's illness, the first difficulty might be to find an appropriate point for the beginning. Just like I started all the other opening interviews, I began the interview with Tony with a rather open question about him being part of the patient school where we first had met.

Example 1 (Names of people and places in the examples have been changed.)

1	PB:	/ . . . / what I'm a bit curios about, it is you and your problems, and how it happened that you turned up at this clinic ((CFS ward)), and actually attended the patient school. (Tony: mm) would you like to tell me a little about this?
2	(1.2)	
3	Tony:	yeah (0.8) what should I say (1.7) 94, 6 years ago that it started in the autumn.
4	(1.8)	
5		.h yeah hh but the thing is, that I began the patient school a bit late, you might think,
6		because- then I fe- felt quite well, if you compare to how I (have) felt earlier.
7	(1.7)	

(continued)

Example 1 (continued)

8	PB:	you- you felt quite well then?
9	Tony:	during the patient school yes. (PB: °mm°)
10	(1.0)	
11		but- yes compared to what I had felt earlier. (PB: mm)
12	(1.0)	
13		°so° I'm on the right- (0.7) on the right way °anyway.° (PB: °mm°)
14	(1.4)	
15		but it was last autumn (0.5) 99 it was. (0.6) when I was (0.9) tired so I went to the doctor
16	(1.2)	
17		and thought that now, they have to take care of (this).
18	(1.7)	
19		.hh so then he ((the doctor)) sent a referral (0.4) to the hospital then.
20		°so they asked me to come (to) the patient school° (PB: °mm°)
21	(2.1)	
22		eh (1.8) ye:s (1.5) .h you have to- hh ask ((me)) a little

In most other interviews, the invitation to describe how the interviewee came to attend the patient school was met by an extended story. In some cases the interviewee initially showed some hesitation about where to begin the story, usually without further difficulties though. For Tony this request seemed to be more problematic.

The whole part shown in Example 1 in different ways displays the difficulty Tony seemed to have to begin to tell me about his illness. This passage includes a lot of pauses as well as restarts and is partly told in a rather low voice. There are several clearly audible in-breaths (.h) as well as out-breaths (hh) which together, as in lines 5 and 22, give the impression of a sigh, as if he finds the task very difficult. These things contribute to the impression of a fumbling and stumbling beginning of the storytelling.

What also makes the beginning of the story "broken" is that each clause is told separately. Different scholars provide various answers to the question of how to define a story. However, most of them probably agree that temporality and coherence are crucial for regarding something as a story. Stories are commonly considered to concern the past. But more important is the temporal ordering, that a story concerns something that happens and changes. According to Riessman and Quinney (2005), it is sequence and consequence that distinguish narrative from other forms of discourse. In a similar way, Carroll (2001) argues that causation defines the narrative connection. By connecting different parts of a "text" in a meaningful way stories are built. They become coherent. For social linguistics the structure defines a story. Probably the most cited person is William Labov (1972; Labov & Waletzky, 1967). According to Labov, the oral narrative of personal experiences includes six elements (if fully formed): abstract, orientation, complicated action, evaluation, result or resolution and, finally, coda. This structure emphasizes the temporal arrangement between different clauses and the chronological formation. Labov defines narrative as "one method of recapitulating past experience by matching a verbal sequence of clauses to the sequence of events which (it is inferred) actually occurred" (Labov, 1972, pp. 359–360).

In the example above, it is possible to identify three different parts: the beginning of illness (line 3), to which Tony gave a rather distinct start; his account of beginning the patient school late—in relation to how he felt "then" as well as how he regarded illness at the time of the interview (lines 5–13); and, finally, the events that preceded his participation in the patient school (lines 15–20). All three parts were accounted for in a rather clear way but with quite few words and without clear combining links between them and the different times mentioned in each part. As individual parts and according to structural definitions about what a story is, only the third can be judged as a *story* including agents and actions. The other two are more like statements or descriptions of something which might have turned into a story but did not, as if he started a story at one point and after some thoughts about what he just said, picked up another thread, starting a new story at another point of time. Finally, Tony's explicit wish to be guided by questions indicates the problem he seems to have to begin to tell a story about his illness.

When I much later tried to understand why the interviews with Tony appeared to me as troublesome and as broken narratives, his repeated wish for me asking him questions seemed important. It was as if he needed some kind of "hooks" to "hang" different experiences and events upon to sort out and to shape a story about his illness.

In a participation/observation study, Dunning (1985) discusses the difference between a reluctant and a willing storyteller in the classroom. During a story-telling session, one boy, who had been absent for a short period of time due to a minor medical operation, was asked to contribute with a story about his time in the hospital. He was reluctant and accepted only if he could "just sit there and you can ask me questions" (Dunning, 1985, p. 2). After some time of questioning and stumbling storytelling, the boy seemed to start to interact with the audience (his classmates) and was no longer dependent on the questions from his teachers. This storytelling was followed by a girl who volunteered for a story about staying in the hospital. This story, which is described as an "unbroken narrative" (p. 7), was very long and more like a monologue (and similar to the Labovian story), hardly ever interrupted by the class. Dunning argues that the difference between these two storytellers depends on the context of the stories, that the boy "came into possession of his story during the course of the lesson" whereas the girl "had arrived ready equipped" (p. 6).

> In David's case, it was clear enough that this context-dialogue was the one we were currently engaged in with him in the classroom. In Kerry's case, however, the context-dialogue consisted of all the talk there had been on the subject over the preceding six years. She came to the lesson with an already prepared report, as it were. (Dunning, 1985, p. 6)

In relation to Dunning's findings it is interesting that Kirmayer (2000) notes that in acute illness, narratives are often fragmentary or undeveloped and that prior to narratives, metaphors can express illness experiences. Inversely, Kirmayer means that most coherent narratives may be "formulaic and distant from sufferers' experience" (2000, p. 153). Even though Tony had been ill for many years, he seemed to be unaccustomed to narrativizing his experience. This can explain why the story is tentative rather than formulaic and stabilized, which many other stories in my material seemed to be. Even if he was never reluctant to answer, Tony, just as the boy in Dunning's study, explicitly asked for guidance by questions.

COCONSTRUCTING THE BEGINNING OF STORYTELLING

Contrary to the narrative structure Labov and Waletzky (1967) plead for, another line of researchers claim coherence to appear in interaction between storyteller and audience or, perhaps more correctly, conarrators. What becomes meaningful and heard as a story is a joint achievement grounded in the "context of practice and the cultural fabric of meaning within which the narrative event takes place," writes Brockmeier (2005, p. 309). Mishler (1999) argues that all sorts of principles and rules to distinguish what makes something a coherent story or not in the end "boils down to the notion that if we can 'make sense' of a passage—any kind of sense—it is *ipso facto* coherent" (p. 84, italics in original). This means that coherence is not to be found "in the text" but interactionally achieved "produced through and embedded in the dialogue" (p. 110). According to Mishler, this process of making sense continues into the analysis of an interview. Following this line, it is interesting in what way Tony and I during the interview jointly tried to shape a story that made sense for both of us.

As shown in Example 2 below, I obviously noticed Tony's problems with finding a way to start telling me about his experiences. It seems to me now as if I was anxious to support him and that I started to formulate a question even before he concluded his request. Taking up one of the time-markers he used, I tried to get him back to the story he seemed to begin a moment ago by saying: "94 you said?"

Example 2

1	Tony:	eh (1.8) ye:s (1.5) .h you have to- hh [ask ((me)) a little
2	PB	[yes
3		.h so [94 you said?
4	Tony:	[cause this is- I (have) trie- ye:s
5	PB:	then you began to feel?
6	Tony:	yes it was dan- you know this .h I should have been on sick leave then. *then.*
7		but then you are too weak, and (0.5) sick to take- to have the strength to take care of things (PB: °yes°)
8		so it- every- everything was just a vicious circle
9		those were (0.5) horrible years. (1.6) in my life.
10	(0.3)	
11	PB:	cou- start with that part. how was it? how did you notice this? wh- in what way?
12	(2.1)	
13	Tony:	yeah (1.3) yes but it started it it ye:ah (0.5) several factors. ((exhaling)) hh
14	(1.2)	
15		well I began at the university ((he starts to tell me about what his life looked like 6 years back in time.))
/.../		
38	Tony:	.hh and *then* all the problems started to come hh (1.0) °after that°.
39		yes in the middle of that semester 94. (1.0) I became sick.
40	(1.3)	
41		Several times in a row.

Jointly, we tried to find a way to start and Tony began to describe what his life looked like when the illness started. At first, in general terms and later—after my specific request—by telling me what happened 6 years ago. He mentioned a number of events that preceded his fatigue—embarking on university studies (as the first member of his family), breaking up with his girlfriend, flunking an examination—all of these were presented as "factors" that he thought might explain why he became ill. It was a chronologically presented story of few words told in a telegraphic style. Short narrative clauses were mixed with evaluations, accounts about what could have happened and side-tracks as well as pauses.

One interesting detail in the example above is the way Tony concluded this part of his story by repeating the time "in the middle of that semester 94" (line 39) that I used in my question (line 3). By doing this, he seemed to make sure that I got the story "right." This shows that the context of this story is the dialogue between Tony and me.

This marked conarrating was not only part of the beginning of the first interview. On the contrary, Tony's explicit wish to be guided by questions and my efforts to make it easier for him influenced the interview as a whole (and the two following interviews). When he stopped, sometimes in the middle of what I understood as a story about something important to Tony, I tried to ask him a follow-up question, or encouraged him in other ways to continue by echoing the last thing he was saying, asking things like "what happened then?" or providing sum-ups like "so this was 1995?" and so forth. Tony often oriented the story in time and perhaps since he was a student at the beginning of his illness he used terms, courses, and exams as the most common points to mark time ("the next ten-point course," "now then we are at the spring term 95 then . . ."). As a result, the story of Tony's illness developed during the interview and it became chronologically quite easy to follow, moving forward from spring to autumn year after year. Our mutual use of time-markers was probably of great importance in telling the story as well as "the following of the story" as Ricoeur (1981) calls the counter part of storytelling. At the same time, the frequent use of time-markers indicates the tentative form of the story and that Tony was searching back in time while he was talking. He seemed to use the chronological form to remember as well as to organize his remembrances into a story. And we both used the same time-markers to orient ourselves in what was told and to go on with a story, which made sense.

SIGNS OF BROKENNESS

Compared to other interviewees in the study, Tony made a lot of comments about the interview and the current situation. At times, when he seemed to have problems narrating his experiences, he commented this with words like: "what difficult questions you ask" or "I don't know what to say," and when he sometimes spontaneously added things, he made comments like "I forgot to say that but . . ." or "and that I've not said either." Besides his actual words, he frequently gave short laughs, which I understood as signs of embarrassment. Even by the way he moved his body I could tell that he felt unease with the situation. He often changed his body position with a sudden movement like throwing himself backwards in the chair. On the tape one could hear the sound of scraping feet. All this gave me the impression that he was uncomfortable with the situation and a feeling that he was not used to talking about his illness in this way.

Just like Tony, I made comments about the situation. More than in other interviews, I could hear myself suggesting interpretations and asking Tony if this was what he meant. Primarily, this was because I had a problem following the story. Sometimes Tony restarted his storytelling at the beginning of these kinds of follow-up questions and comments, or even at the same time as if my act of speaking rather than my words pushed him to continue (see Example 2, lines 3–4). As a result, there was more overlapping talk in this interview than in most others.

When I much later returned to the tapes and retranscribed these interviews I realized that the *brokenness* I experienced during the interviews was also noticeable in the text in the way Tony told short, fragmented, and uncompleted stories, which almost never were concluded by a resolution or by a coda (Labov & Waletzky, 1967). Instead, most of his stories just ended by a sharp cut-off or he left them unfinished in a lower voice as shown in Example 3 below.

Example 3

1	Tony:	so I had to borrow money there from my friends (0.5) that autumn
2		so when the course ended I had twenty-five thousand in debt to my friends instead
3		so one got another stress factor that became a burden. (PB: °mm°)
4		°which one maybe didn't (.) feel so good because of really°
5		cause I had this debt with me for two years or so °I had that before I got rid of it°
6	(3.0)	
7		°yes°
8	(2.0)	
9	PB:	but that was in the autumn 96. then you were studying again
10	Tony:	yes then it was full-time (°again.°) (PB: °mm°)
11		it went on quite well that course °then°
12	(1.0)	
13		.hhh yes hh then where were we then?
14		°spring semester 97 what was it then?°
15	(4.5)	
16		°I rem- yeah that's right then I took it a a little easy for (a while)°
17		°then I took- ((studied on his own)) (0.8) (a) course there°
18	(4.3)	

Example 3 (continued)

19		part-time then °one could say.°
20	(3.2)	
21		°yes:°
22	(1.4)	
23		°I don't rem- you know the years become a bit mixed up° ((gives a short quiet laugh))
24	PB:	but what was it that made ((you)) that it was just- (.) that it was eh what was it that made you start seeing a doctor in 99?
25	Tony:	yeah one can wonder about that.
26		YES BUT THAT- THAT IN SOME WAY- (1.2) one went on all the time thinking like this "this will stop" (PB: yes) "this will stop."
27		yes so- and then ((I)) fe- had felt- some day when one felt a little better
28		one felt like this "now (it's) going to be alright" (PB: °mm°)
29	(0.7)	
30		((swallows))
31	(0.8)	
32		((gives a short laugh)) *and that-* that I've been reminded about that by my sister.
33		.hh °she (has-)° .h always complained hh that I should seek help from- psychiatric care in some way
34		°(and) talk to a- (.) psychologist or something.°

The pattern that appears in Example 3 was in many ways typical for the interviews with Tony with its shift in perspectives—stressed by a shift in pronouns from "I" to "one"—sudden transitions and endings of stories as well as the variation of strength in his voice. When relistening to the tape recordings, I found that Tony's voice was loud and clear when starting to say something but then shortly after losing both speed and strength, turning into almost a whisper. Sometimes, like in lines 13–21 in Example 3, it was like he was talking to himself rather than me. This variation of voice becomes very clear in the last part of the example above (lines 26–28) when he begins to tell the story of why he went to the doctor in 1999, 5 years after his illness began.

A reasonable question is if this pattern had something to do with Tony's and my different expectations of the interview: him waiting for questions to orient to and myself expecting narratives. In that case, the troublesome storytelling is basically a methodological problem.

The narrative turn within social science—including life stories and illness narratives which started about two decades ago—has had a great impact on studies of illness experience perspective (Bell, 2000). Today, researchers—not only within social science but within humanities and medicine as well—are actually looking for illness narratives and for how ill persons narrativize their experience. This turn in perspectives has also changed many researchers' ideas about interviewing people—which is probably the most common way to elicit stories of life. Riessman (2001) reminds us how most social scientists not very long ago made a lot of efforts to formulate questions leading to as short and clear-cut answers as possible from their respondents. Today, it is more likely to be the other way around—that many researchers encourage interviewees to tell their stories about whatever is the issue of the study. Thus, framing the interview situation in such a way that it will evoke stories as elaborated as possible has become important. It is not certain, however, whether the interviewees always are prepared for this emphasis on storied experiences. On this issue, Mishler (1986) argues that it is most likely to get stories as answers even to rather narrow questions and that the absence of narratives in research interviews can be explained by researchers interrupting their interviewees or neglecting stories in their analysis. Accordingly, what a researcher hears and counts as a story becomes important for the results of the studies. Perhaps the difficulty I assumed Tony had in telling me about his illness was not only connected to what each of us was expecting from the interview, but also had to do with my view of stories. If I had been waiting for more well-defined stories, like the Labovian ones, then the scanty narrating of Tony might appear as broken narratives. But were they really "broken"?

RETELLING THE "UNTOLD" STORIES

Analysing the interviews with Tony revealed that what at first thought seemed to be broken narratives later turned out to be a lot of story fragments that were unfinished, undeveloped, and interrupted. Yet those fragments disclosed much about suffering from a contested illness. Nevertheless, the broken manner of Tony's storytelling, the "unfinished" stories and shifts in perspectives——which continued even in longer episodes of telling——the pauses, comments, and the way his voice seemed to lose its strength increased my impression of a tentative story that was created there and then. This story, in great parts, was previously untold, maybe even to himself. This was partly confirmed by Tony, who said that he had not actually told anyone about his illness before he went to the patient school. On occasions when his fatigue had become visible to other people, like when he was bird watching with a friend and had to lay down on the ground, he did not explain the reason for his doings. That the story of his illness probably was more or less "untold" before the interviews might explain the broken manner of storytelling. But if so, stories that recurred in the interviews could be expected to change just as the boy's storytelling in Dunning's (1985) study. And they did. Already at the end of the first interview, Tony summarized the part of the story of why he became ill. When I met him for a second interview about half a year later and asked him what he thought about this kind of illness, he once more told me the story of what caused his illness.

Example 4

1	PB:	/ . . . / but what do you think yourself that such fatigue comes from?
2	Tony:	yes but there were many factors involved *then*. (2.0) really.
3	(2.0)	
4		it was- (1.7) in the autumn 94 when everything happened in some way °like I said° (PB: °yes°)
5		started at the university, broke up with my girlfriend, and I became ill all the time.
6		obviously it was- I don't know- ME ((CFS)) or not I still don't know if I have had that or not.
7	(1.0)	
8		but according to Xxx ((the medical specialist)) it really was- a virus can trigger-
9		cause I remember I had some nasty infections you know. (0.5) with fever and- (0.5) things
10	(0.8)	
11		and then after that I was never well.
12	(3.5)	
13		yes then there was stress involved too. (0.5) so it became.
14	(1.0)	
15		°and so I failed exams and,°
16	(1.5)	
17		yeah high ambitions when one started studying. ((at the university))
18	(3.5)	
19		so it was I guess something that happened there. (0.5) that has stayed that way.
20	(3.0)	
21		then eh (0.8) I think that it's a pity that I maybe should have given up there like I've said before.
22	PB	°mm yes you've said that yes°
23	(1.0)	
24	Tony:	not struggle and struggle struggle °struggle°

Compared to the story he told 6 months earlier, this one seemed to be more fluent. Not in the sense that it was more elaborated, which was not the case, but because it appeared as a story that had been told a sufficient number of times to turn it into a "short version." Tony also explicitly referred to having told me this before ("like I said" in lines 4 and 21). Still with lots of pauses and with quite few words, this version contained the same elements as the story about becoming ill told in the opening interview and was temporally organised in a similar way. The main difference was that the story this time had been condensed. Instead of telling short stories about each "factor"—starting university, breaking up with his girlfriend, failing examinations and becoming ill—he presented these as key events in lines 5, 15, and 17. The marked pauses between almost every single clause made them even more clearly appear as keywords which together form a core narrative. In line 19 he concluded the story with a resolution that linked up what happened, and the hypothetical thought about sick leave in the earlier story (Example 2, line 6) now appeared at the end as postscript (lines 21 and 24). The difference between the two versions indicates that the broken manner is not just a personal style of storytelling but rather the consequence of a previously "untold" story—or seldom narrated experience.

STORIES ABOUT REJECTED STORIES

The difficulty in telling others about his illness was also part of the content of the stories told. During the interviews, Tony described four meetings with different physicians. In three of these encounters, his suffering and his story about it seemed to have been rejected. The first time he went to see a doctor because of the fatigue happened when Tony had been ill for about 1 year. The story about this occasion was told quite some time into the first interview.

Example 5

1	PB:	.h when you looked for help (.) so then when you asked for help from the health care 99-
2	Tony:	mm but I must say that I did- I forgot to tell you that ((before)) but I did seek ((help)) 95 in the autumn the first time.
3		Then I sought help (.) at the local health care centre
4		(and) they did some tests
5		and I was healthy.
6	(.)	
7	PB:	You went there and said that you didn't feel well or?
8	Tony:	Yeah. Yes (.) tired and sick all the time I said (.)°something like that°

(continued)

Example 5 (continued)

9	and (.) cause it's like that you tried to find a physical reason kind of
10	.h but the tests were alright
11	And then I thought that it could be some kind of allergy maybe I thought that too.
12	Had an allergy test
13	That was perfectly alright too.
14	So he told me that it is all in the head (.) said the doctor
15	Yes (.) so you left
16	Then it took 4 years before I sought help next time.

In this story we can, as listeners and readers, only imagine how Tony tried to explain his experience to the doctor. As a response to my suggestion about what he might have said in the encounter (line 7) he retold a tiny part of the dialogue but left most of it unspoken. Yet, from Tony's reflections on this meeting it is quite easy to fill in and to visualize what might have happened when the first tests did not indicate any kind of disease and how Tony continued to claim feeling ill. Might it perhaps be allergy? What becomes perfectly clear is how the doctor rejected the story Tony told him by explaining Tony's problems as something "all in the head" (line 14) and thus imagination. This leaves Tony's story without credibility and the suffering as *delegitimated* to use one of Ware's (1992) concepts. As a consequence, his story was silenced since he avoided this kind of situation for many years.

What is also interesting is how Tony seemed to recollect this episode when asked about another more recent medical encounter, which he had already briefly mentioned. It is as the experience of rejection itself has been rejected but recalled in the context of the interview. The first minimal narrative (lines 3–5) about the medical encounter supports this interpretation. According to Linde (1993), such narratives are extremely rare but seem to occur in situations when "the speaker is for some reason obliged to tell a narrative that is unpleasant or painful to recount" (p. 69). However, the two episodes are connected since this first contact with the health care system, due to CFS, explains why it took 4 more years of suffering before Tony decided to visit another physician. This story then brings both consequence and sequence to the first one told at the beginning of the interview (Example 1) about receiving a referral to the hospital and a specialist. Once more, the scanty storytelling seems to be part of a narrative in progress.

Tony told me about two other times when different doctors rejected his story in various ways. One of these occurred 4 years after his first try (Example 5) when his complaint was met with a prescription for nose drops. The next time the specialist simply did not regard him as suffering from CFS. According to the specialist, Tony met three of the needed four criteria to receive the diagnosis. Tony commented this judgement with the words "but I saw that I fulfilled more." Not only physicians rejected Tony's stories. When he could not keep the pace with the required number of study credits at the university, he wrote a letter to the national authority that handles the financial aid for students, asking to be allowed to keep his grants and to continue receiving his loans. His request was turned down. Instead he had to borrow money from his friends (see Example 3) and later take a pause in his university studies.

All these times when Tony had tried to tell physicians and officials about his illness without being heard probably affected his willingness to talk about his illness. From stories about avoiding telling anyone about how he felt, untold or tacit stories emerged. Even when his fatigue became obvious, like in bird watching, he refrained from explaining it (see page 14). When asked how he explained his situation to family and friends, he usually answered that he never told anyone about illness.

Example 6

1	PB:	What did you say to people when you- when they well said "come on" ((join us))
2	Tony:	°oh° (I) don't have the strength
3	(.)	
4	PB:	How was that received?
5	Tony:	Well (.) it is well that kind of things they accepted it probably
6		but they never got any explanation.
7		The guy that I- that I was studying together with during my first year ((at university)) actually when I studied in 94
8		He and I were both single then and would go out and have some-
9		yeah he phoned quite often then
10		but I have never told him anything until now this fall it was ((laughs))
11		Why?
12	(.)	
13	PB:	Why you told him now this fall ((you mean))?
14	Tony:	No but you know I said s- explained why I couldn't do things
15	PB:	Yes, right 94
16	Tony:	yeah, (I) explained it now ((year)) two thousand ((laughs))

(continued)

Example 6 (continued)

17	PB:	yes
18	Tony:	mhm
19	PB:	Did he understand that or had he guessed something or?
20	Tony:	No, no but I conf- you confessed then.
21		I don't know (what he thought)
22		Cause if people ask how you're doing one says "well" like
23		Yes, but it's different if one has gotten cancer or something
24		(then) one would maybe say that ((laughs))
25		but this- this is so .h I haven't really understood what it is you know that I have come up against something
26		But now I haven't received the diagnosis of CFS but
27	(.)	
28	PB:	Yes, you said so
29	Tony:	.hh ((clears his throat)) but I'm well pretty sure that it is that ((CFS)) or-
30		yes some symptoms have disappeared after all so something happened
31	(.)	

Being reluctant to tell his friends about his illness and what made it difficult for him to join them for various activities seemed to be connected to the difficulty to describe an illness like CFS. Tony's comparison with suffering from cancer indicates such a view. However, his experiences of rejected stories in encounters with physicians also seem to be part of this choice to avoid talking about fatigue in other situations as well, since the lack of a diagnosis have made him uncertain about what it is he is suffering from (lines 25–26). Even if he is "pretty sure" (line 29) none of his physicians have confirmed that it is CFS he suffers from.

As stated in the beginning, to tell someone about a contested illness means to take a risk. Later in the first interview, when I returned to the question about how he explained his illness today, Tony gave another example of disclosing (Example 7).

Since fatigue is a common feeling, it can be difficult to recognize it as illness even for the ill person himself or herself. To claim then that this ordinary feeling is chronic and part of a diagnosis is even more complicated. Instead of functioning as an explanation for certain behavior, like not having the strength to keep up with work, friends, or the pace of study, disclosing fatigue often results in what Ware (1992) calls *trivialisation* of the experience. When everyone can say "I am also tired all the time" then those suffering from CFS run the risk of being called into question. For

Example 7

1	Tony:	((laughs)) if I tell (you)
2		I told one guy in my new class today that I was going to see you here
3		But then the reaction is like that (.) you are a bit afraid of starting to talk about it
4		cause people know fatigue everybody feels it.
5	(.)	
6		So he said that today too "I might also have that" eh like that
7	(.)	
8		°It feels like it's no use going into details. No I simply can't°

some sufferers this might lead to restrictions on narrating one's experience and to fewer stories due to stigmatization, morality, contestation, or uncertainty about legitimacy. However, what is really interesting in this story—and the one in Example 6—is that these narratives describe how Tony recently had started to be more open about his illness. Thus, the presented examples indicate not only a narrative in progress but also the interactive process in which this is happening.

THE PROBLEM OF TROUBLESOME STORYTELLING

In this chapter I have examined what at first appeared to me as broken narratives or, perhaps more correctly described, as an illness narrative presented in a broken manner. By analyzing a series of interviews with a young man suffering from CFS, I have shown how storytelling that seems to be broken differs from what usually is thought of as a typical story. Unlike the range of temporally connected elements (as in the Labovian narrative structure), the examined interviews turned out to consist of a number of minimal narratives and story fragments intersected with pauses and sighs. Besides that, the stories told in such a broken style tended to be more explicitly emanating from the interaction between the young man and me as his interlocutor. The narratives were dialogically told rather then presented as "prepared" stories in the form of a monologue.

I have argued that a possible reason why personal experiences sometimes are told in a broken manner is because such stories concern things that the storyteller seldom or perhaps never before have tried to narrate. I have therefore asserted that it is a matter of *narratives in progress,* that the storyteller during the conversation, through questions and his or her own reasoning, gradually comes into possession of a story of life (cf. Dunning). The broken manner can thus be called broken only in the same way as when a nonnative English speaker speaks in broken English.

The reasons for not being used to put one's experiences into a story can be several. One plausible cause is because what is about to be told happened recently. Another reason, however, which I have been arguing for in this text, is that the storyteller is unaccustomed to narrativizing the experience of long-term illness since he or she finds it too difficult to tell a story about an illness that might be contested, or that the ill person avoids narrating the experience by way of precaution.

Since stories told in a broken manner are strongly depending on interaction, they are always at the peril of being left unnoticed due to difficulties of establishing a joint understanding. In research interviews, such as those I have been examining here, there is an obvious risk that we as researchers pay less attention to broken narratives, leaving them behind, unanalyzed as unimportant and irrelevant material because they do not look like stories are supposed to do, or because they are regarded as less useful examples. Yet, storytelling that seems to be incoherent, or broken may show something important about the experience of illness and even about the medical encounter.

Just as broken narratives can be left unnoticed in research interviews there is a risk that such stories are not taken into consideration during the medical investigation. In a clinical framework Kirmayer (2000, p. 169) identifies a variety of ways that examining the "failure to construct a mutually satisfying joint narrative" breaks narratives. When the medical consultation concerns illnesses like CFS, the need for constructing a jointly satisfying narrative is of great importance since in the end it is in the interaction that diagnosis can be reached. If stories told in a broken manner are not heard as stories—or as stories about a certain illness—this can imply that people who tell a less coherent story will not receive a diagnosis like CFS for which the story is crucial. There are indications that those who are diagnosed to suffer from CFS are rather well-educated (Natelson, 1998), something which might enforce this argument since it is more likely that the physician and the well-educated patient share a certain view of how to tell a convincing story. A story told in a broken way can thus be said to have a lower degree of credibility—and the storyteller to a greater extent comes at risk of becoming contested.

Not receiving a name for one's suffering probably lessens a person's possibility to narrate their illness experience. Lacking a diagnosis (though disputed) often makes it harder to tell trustworthy stories in different situations. Invisible sufferings without a medical label are easy to dismiss. If this lack is connected to, or perhaps the consequence of, a rejected story, the willingness to narrate one's illness is very likely much reduced. Sufferers who have not received a diagnosis may become restrictive in their storytelling and thus unaccustomed to narrativizing their illness. In relation to the idea that often told experiences reach a more fixed and stabilized form, it is of significance that Tony in my examples hardly ever talked about his illness. If it was the difficulty in formulating a narrative that made this man restrictive in telling people about his illness, or if it was because he had rarely told this story—perhaps not even to himself—that led to the brokenness of the narrative analyzed here, to these questions I have no answer. Neither can I tell if it was because of the difficulty in presenting a convincing story that this man did not receive the diagnosis of CFS when he first contacted a doctor—or if the brokenness of his narrating was the consequence of being rejected by the physician and after that becoming restrictive in telling people about his illness.

All these explanations are possible within a view of narratives as a particularly important and powerful resource to make sense of illness and to present ourselves—especially when identity and a sense of self are considered as part of the social context. One additional reason why a man is restrictive in telling about CFS is that it could be more difficult for men to present themselves as suffering from an illness which is described as an illness where about 70% of the sufferers are female. Since none of the women seemed to have any problems in telling their story, but 2 out of 4 men did, this is a possible thought.

Considering the idea about people narratively reconstructing a life story which has been disrupted due to chronic illness (Williams, 1984), those who never or seldom tell people about their experiences might have difficulties in incorporating illness into their story of life. When it comes to contested illnesses like CSF it is important to ask if it is the risk of not being trusted that makes some people restrictive in telling others about their experiences, or if they avoid narrating because illness is hard to describe as a disease. The difficulty in making sense probably worsens if the sufferers do not receive a diagnosis rendering some confirmation. From a narrative perspective, this means difficulties for the ill person in attaching his or her individual experience into the larger story about CFS, thus leading to a continuous search for a diagnosis or concealment of illness.

All this boils down to methodology and the delicate work of analyzing narratives, perhaps especially illness narratives. If we really want to learn as much as possible about living with a certain illness—be it a stigmatizing diagnosis, a contested illness, or a fatal disease—it is of great importance that we carefully examine all kinds of narrating, also those which do not look like stories at first glance. As researchers we must ask ourselves why some people tell stories about their illnesses in a certain way while others do not present us narratives of the illness. Is it because of the interview situation or because of something else? By relistening to and retranscribing recorded material, new interpretations can be made and new questions can be posed and discussed.

Finally, the call for stories, which Frank writes about and which I quoted at the beginning of this chapter, is double-edged when the ill are suffering from a contested illness. As sufferer you need to tell stories about your condition for the possibility of having it confirmed and diagnosed, but at the same time these stories are always at risk of becoming contested. However, it does not stop at this. If being called into question, it seems as if the readiness to tell stories about illness can be affected so that the ill person hesitates to narrate even when we as researchers call for stories.

TRANSCRIPT KEY

(0.5)	pause
(.)	short pause
.hh/hh	audible inbreath/outbreath
(( ))	transcriber's comments or nonverbal activity like
-	sharp cut-off
[	onset of a spate of overlapping talk
(xxx)	inaudible
:	stretching of the preceding sound or letter
(guess)	uncertain interpretation
.	a full stop indicates a stopping fall in tone
,	a comma indicates a 'continuing' intonation
?	a question mark indicates a rising inflection
°quiet°	noticeably quieter than surrounding talk
CAPITALS	speech noticeably louder than surrounding talk
under	*emphasized* word or words
with laugh	with laughter in voice
/ . . . /	passage omitted

REFERENCES

Bell, S. E. (2000). Experiencing illness in/and narrative. In C. E. Bird, P. Conrad, & A. M. Fremont (Eds.), *Handbook of medical sociology* (pp. 184–199). Upper Saddle River, NJ: Prentice Hall.

Brockmeier, J. (2005). Pathways of narrative meaning construction. In G. Bruce D & C. S. Tamis-LeMonda (Eds.), *The development of social cognition and communication* (pp. 291–313). Mahwah, NJ: Lawrence Erlbaum Associates.

Bülow, P. H. (2004). Sharing experiences of contested illness by storytelling. *Discourse & Society, 15,* 33–53.

Bülow, P. H. (2008). Tracing contours of contestation in narratives about chronic fatigue syndrome. In P. Moss & K. Teghtsoonian (Eds.), *Contesting illness: Processes and practice.* Toronto, Canada: University of Toronto Press (pp. 121–141).

152   *Pia Bülow*

Bülow, P. H., & Hydén, L. C. (2003a). In dialogue with time: Identity and illness in narratives about chronic fatigue. *Narrative Inquiry, 13*, 71–97.

Bülow, P. H., & Hydén, L. C. (2003b). Patient school as a Way of creating meaning in contested illness: The case of CFS. *Health: An Interdisciplinary Journal for the Social Study of Health, Illness and Medicine, 7*, 227–249.

Carroll, N. (2001). *Beyond aesthetics: Philosophical essays.* Cambridge, UK: Cambridge University Press.

Dumit, J. (2006). Illnesses you have to fight to get: Facts as forces in uncertain, emergent illnesses. *Social Science & Medicine, 62*, 577–590.

Dunning, J. (1985). Reluctant and willing story tellers in the classroom. *English in Education, 19*, 1–15.

Evengård, B., Schacterle, F. S., & Komaroff, A. L. (1999). Chronic fatigue syndrome: New insights and old ignorance. *Journal of Internal Medicine, 246*, 455–469.

Frank, A. W. (1995). *The wounded storyteller: Body, illness, and ethics.* Chicago: The University of Chicago Press.

Fukuda, K., Straus, S. E., Hickie, I., Sharpe, M., Dobbins, J. G., Komaroff, A., et al. (1994). The chronic fatigue syndrome: A comprehensive approach to its definition and study. *Annals of Internal Medicine, 121*, 953–959.

Good, B. J., & Good, M-J. D. V. (1994). In the subjunctive mode: Epilepsy narratives in Turkey. *Social Science and Medicine, 38*, 835–842.

Holmes, G. P., Kaplan, J. E., Gantz, N. M., Komaroff, A. L., Schonberger, L. B., Straus, S. E., et al. (1988). Chronic fatigue syndrome: A working case definition. *Annals of Internal Medicine, 108*, 387–389.

Hydén, L. C. (1997). Illness and narrative. *Sociology of Health & Illness, 19*(7), 48–69.

Hydén, L. C., & Bulow, P. (2006). Medical discourse, Illness narratives. In K. Brown (Ed.), *Encyclopedia of language and linguistics, 2nd Ed.* (Vol. 7, pp. 697–703). Oxford, UK: Elsivier.

Hydén, L. C., & Sachs, L. (1998). Suffering, hope and diagnosis: On the negotiation of chronic fatigue syndrome. *Health, 2*, 175–193.

Joyce, J., Hotopf, M., & Wessely, S. (1997). The prognosis of chronic fatigue and chronic fatigue syndrome: A systematic review. *The Quarterly Journal of Medicine, 90*, 223–233.

Kirmayer, L. J. (2000). Broken narratives: Clinical encounters and the poetics of illness experience. In C. Mattingly & L. C. Garro (Eds.), *Narrative and the cultural construction of illness and healing* (pp. 153–180). London: University of California Press.

Labov, W. (1972). The transformation of experience in narrative syntax. In W. Labov (Ed.), *Language in the inner city* (pp. 354–405). Philadelphia: University of Pennsylvania Press.

Labov, W., & Waletzky, J. (1967). Narrative analysis: Oral versions of personal experience. In J. Helm (Ed.), *Essays on the verbal and visual arts* (pp. 12–44). Seattle, WA: University of Washington Press.

Linde, C. (1993). *Life stories: The creation of coherence.* Oxford, UK: Oxford University Press.

Mishler, E. G. (1986). *Research interviewing: Context and narrative.* Cambridge, MA: Harvard University Press.

Mishler, E. G. (1999). *Storylines: Craftartists' narratives of identity.* Cambridge, MA: Harvard University Press.

Natelson, B. H. (1998). *Facing and fighting fatigue: A practical approach.* New Haven, CT: Yale University Press.

Rabinbach, A. (1992). *The Human motor: Energy, fatigue, and the origins of modernity.* Berkeley, CA: University of California Press.

Ricoeur, P. (1981). Narrative time. In W. J. T. Mitchell (Ed.), *On narrative* (pp. 165–186). Chicago: The University of Chicago Press.

Riessman, C. K. (2001). Analysis of personal narratives. In J. F. Gubrium & J. A. Holstein (Eds.), *Handbook of interview research: Context & method* (pp. 695–710). Thousand Oaks, CA: Sage.

Riessman, C. K., & Quinney, L. (2005). Narrative in social work: A critical review. *Qualitative Social Work, 4,* 391–412.

Ware, N. C. (1992). Suffering and the social construction of illness: The delegitimation of illness experience in chronic fatigue syndrome. *Medical Anthropology Quarterly, 4,* 347–361.

Ware, N. C., & Kleinman, A. (1992). Culture and somatic experience: The social course of illness in neurasthenia and chronic fatigue syndrome. *Psychosomatic Medicine, 54,* 546–560.

Williams, G. H. (1984). The genesis of chronic illness: Narrative re-construction. *Sociology of Health and Illness, 6,* 175–200.

9   Break-Up Narratives

Margareta Hydén

This chapter deals with a certain kind of stories of personal experience. I have named them "break-up narratives"—stories people tell and live that offer a basis for identity (re)formation in times of self-inflicted change. I explore the stories women have told me after leaving their abusive men. This exploration keeps me on the same route of inquiry that I have followed for more than 20 years (c.f. Hydén 1994; Hydén & McCarthy, 1994; Hydén 1999; Hydén 2005; Hydén, 2008). Along the way, I have sought answers to questions such as: How do women and men make sense of acts of marital woman battering? How do they define, interpret, and explain these acts? What does violence do to their lives and marriages? When and how do they separate?

Generally speaking, breaking up is about *difference* and *movement*. When you break up, you stage discontinuity in time and location/space. You leave; you depart from something or someone. When a battered woman leaves her husband, she leaves their joint home. At the same time as she changes location, she changes her social space. This self-inflicted disruption, this difference she has administered to herself, gives her opportunities to (re)form her life history. The break-up narrative, I argue, plays an important part in determining along what lines her (re)formed life history can be developed.

The chapter traces its origin to a study of battered women's experiences and demands for help. I selected a group of 10 women and interviewed them on six separate occasions over a 2-year period. The first interview took place at the women's shelter 1 or 2 weeks after the women arrived. Subsequent interviews took place in the women's homes at about 4-month intervals. All the women had been subjected to repeated and serious violence in their marriages. Serious violence is defined as violent actions, for example, kicks, punches, threats with a weapon, attempts to strangle, rape, attempts to rape, etc. Repeated violence means violence that is so frequent that it becomes an integral part of marital life. The group was subject to the shelter's entry criteria and conditions. For example, women with substance abuse problems were not admitted.

Prior to the first interview, I prepared only two questions: "Why did you leave the marriage at this point?" and "What is your life like right now, what is most central to your life right now?" With my opening question, "Why did you leave your marriage at this point," I had expected to get the beginning of the break-up story. I did not. I rather got parts of the middle. Or, I got something that marked the end of something in the woman's mind—and in the process of telling was revealed as one of the many parts that formed the middle of the break-up story. In the course of my investigation, it was pointed out that what was defined as the beginning, middle, and end of the break-up constituted a much more complex pattern. Time was not linear. The events that built up the break-up narrative were not heading in one single direction. The same event could constitute the end of one part of the story and the beginning of the next—and at the same time serve as part of the middle. The same event could be shadowed by time from the future, as well as from the past and the present, and be rendered different meaning, accordingly.

Having now completed my introductory remarks, I go on to tell about battered women's break-up narratives from the beginning. *My* beginning.

NARRATIVE PRE-CONSTRUCTION

About 10 years ago, I was engaged part-time as a psychotherapist at a Battered Women's Shelter in Stockholm, Sweden. One steamy hot day in July, I heard a discreet knock at my door. When I opened, a slender female body was sharply outlined against the light. We had met before at the general meetings on Thursdays. Her name was Maria. She was 34 and the mother of a 10-year-old son.

> **Maria:** May I?
> **Margareta:** Of course, please come in.

Maria had stayed at the shelter for about a month, after having left her abusive husband. Now she sat in front of me with a thin, well-worn notebook in her lap.

> **Maria:** Well, you know, life here gives you time to think and time to share your thoughts with others.
> **Margareta:** Hmm.
> **Maria:** We have talked a great deal about it, we women who are staying here right now. At first, everything is in such a mess. You are so scared, so confused. Fear strikes you, so you are almost paralyzed. All you think of is his revenge. The world outside expects you to be relieved, happy even, while you yourself are mostly pained, tormented. It is a very unpleasant experience; to say the least, do you see what I mean . . . ?
> **Margareta:** Yes, I think so. You are talking about difference, different understandings?

Maria: Yes, and it is painful, because you cannot share your feelings with those outside, those who are happy on your behalf and expect you to be the same. Painful, because when you are in it, in this "state" or whatever you can call it, you think it will last forever. You think you are condemned to spend the rest of your life in confusion and fear. You think you have been broken or something. Broken, once and for all, destroyed. It is unbearable. It brings you almost to the brink of suicide. But the fantastic thing is, it does not last forever, this "state" or what I shall call it? It is just a phase you go thorough. You go on. You continue living. You enter new "states." The problem is that that you don't know that this is just a phase when you are in it This . . . that it is not yet written about . . . that could be changed . . . couldn't it?

Margareta: I imagine so.

Maria: We have begun to write some of it down . . . we would like to share it with you . . . we thought you might be interested. You are doing research and writing about violence towards women, right? Maybe you would like to do some research on it?

I was moved by her sincere request and her confidence in me, at the same time as I was fully aware of the fact that she made great demands on me. What she and the other women would engage me in was not in the writing of *any* kind of break-up story, but a specific one, namely one with the power to heal, a story that they could live with. I knew that Maria was not a "naïve narrator" in the sense that she thought that there was a single and straightforward link between speaking trauma and personal healing. Quite the contrary, she knew that talking about what had happened and healing was a complex one and that taking part in sharing activities as traumatized could even be (re)traumatizing. Her awareness put some fresh courage into me: She knew, that when she asked me to share her story of leaving her abusive man, she knew that what she asked was not only to share the content, but the sensitivity that was carried with it (cf. Hydén, 2008). Upon due consideration, I accepted her invitation. Thus began a 2-year journey of repeated interviewing of 10 women, who had all been subjected to repeated and serious violence in their marriages, left their abusive men, and sought refuge at a shelter for battered women in Stockholm, Sweden. During the course of the 2 years, they left the shelter and created new homes.

"Before a narrative can be constructed, it must be pre-constructed by a cognitive process that begins with a decision that a given event is reportable," William Labov (2006, p. 37) suggests, and continues "pre-construction begins with this most reportable event and proceeds backwards in time to locate events that are linked causally each to the following one." I think what I described above could be described as the pre-construction of my narrative about the battered women's break-up narratives.

A Battered Women's Shelter in Stockholm is a special place in that it offers housing and support for women in exile after they leave abusive relationships. In doing so, it offers social space for all kinds of practices aimed at liberating women from an oppressive man and a patriarchal society. Maria knew this. So when she invited me to take part in a narrative practice she called "research on battered women's break-ups," she knew that she was referring to a category of "events" that had "general reportability" at the shelter.

I agree with Labov that before a narrative can be constructed, a decision has to be made as to whether or not the event is reportable. I disagree, however, with the argument that the decision making always takes the form of a cognitive process. My decision to accept Maria's invitation did include an evaluation of the reportability of the events she and the other women wanted to tell me—it was already considered reportable within the social space that we shared. When I agreed to enter the shelter in my capacity as psychotherapist, I also agreed to give battered women's break-up stories the highest degree of reportability. Further, Maria also knew my research interest—practiced in another social space than the shelter. My work was represented in the shelter's library and discussed among the women. So when she expected me to join her and the other women in their endeavor, this expectation was well founded.

BREAK-UPS AS LIVED EXPERIENCE AND
BREAK-UPS AS NARRATIVE

From my previous research, I had found the same discrepancies Maria was telling me about: In the eyes of others, a break-up from a violent marriage is generally conceived as a single event, composing the demarcation line between "the past evil—and the future good life." Described this way, the break-up experience does not leave much room for agony and pain, but only for joy and celebration of the new opportunities waiting to be staged. Maria's story went in the opposite direction. She told me that the personal experience of the battered woman's break-up constitutes a seemingly endless process characterized by undifferentiated fear that completely overwhelms the woman. This feeling was very difficult to deal with. What had made a recent difference, however, was that she had observed that the totality of her own fear had been reduced and been transformed into something she described as distinguished and more manageable "phases." This alteration brought hope of reaching an end to the painful break-up process—and not *any* end, but a happy one. "Happy" basically meant a life without fear.

I understood Maria's decision to approach me as a way of trying to secure this hope and to take it a bit further. She needed my help to understand her observation as a message from the future that better times were on their way. From what I knew of her, she did not understand this message as a "prophetic sign"—she was a much too down-to-earth person for that. I think she understood her message from the future as encouragement not to give up. I understood her request: "Help us to write down the battered woman's break-up process" as a way of coming to meet the future. By structuring the break-up process in narrative form, she could escape the experience of time as an open field of possibilities, where each element had a set of possible events in which she could participate. Before she had actually left her husband this open time field full of possibilities had brought hope—now it brought quite the contrary, because some of the events that could happen were threatening. Now she wanted to single out one event from this open time field—that of more controlled fear—and base her break-up narrative on it. Worded in that way, the break-up narrative could carry hope and even forebode a happy future.

CLOSE THE TIME FOR ME, PLEASE

Literary historians Michael Bernstein and Gary Morson (1994) have examined the relation of time to narrative form, arguing that it is misleading to assume a single temporality for all disciplines and all aspects of experience. Morson (1994, p. 3) asks: "Might it not be the case that we need multiple concepts of time for diverse purposes and circumstances?" Time can "shadow" the narrative in different ways. Various kinds of *sideshadowing* offer a world in which *time is open*. Sideshadowing admits the presence of real possibilities that could have happened even if they did not. Things could have been different from the way they were; there were real alternatives to the way things turned out to be. By contrast, *foreshadowing* offers a world in which *time is closed*. When foreshadowing is used, certain events take place in a special way. Instead of being caused by prior events, they happen as a consequence of events to come. Foreshadowing, in short, involves backward causation, which means that the future must already be there, must somehow already exist substantially enough to send signs backward (Morson, 1994, p. 7). In addition to sideshadowing and foreshadowing, there is a third "shadow of time," *backshadowing*. Backshadowing is a kind of reactive foreshadowing in which the shared knowledge of the outcome of a series of events by narrator and listener is used to judge their participation in those events as though they should have known what was to come. The past is treated as if it had inevitably to lead to the present we know and as if signs of our present should have been visible to our predecessors (Morson, 1994, p. 13).

"Close the time for me, please, around a predictable and brighter future" is, I think, what Maria was asking me in our first encounter. The way Gary Morson talks about foreshadowing could serve an answer to her prayers:

Foreshadowing robs a present moment of its presentness. Foreshadowing lifts its veil on a future that has already been determined and inscribed. Somehow, a specific later event is already given at the time of an earlier event. What will be must be; events are heading in a single direction; time is entirely linear, because the future is either known for certain or calculable (at least in principle). Wisdom in such a world consists in the appreciation of inevitability. (Morson, 1994, p. 117)

"Please rob this present moment of its presentness," I think Maria was saying to me. "Wisdom in my world consists in the appreciation of inevitability. Please join me in my world and we will both become a bit wiser." But what would such involvement mean? She didn't know the future of her story and neither did I—but I wanted to assist her in telling *her* story, I did not want her to echo my storytelling. So before I started my interviews with Maria, I had to reflect a bit over what degree of involvement would be appropriate.

As noted by Elinor Ochs and Lisa Capps (2001), listeners vary their involvement in the actual telling of a narrative from cursory displays of attentiveness to posing probing questions to supplying narrative details. Relatively high involvement characterizes narrative interaction in which, although one person may be positioned as primary teller, substantive narrative contributions are made by more than one interlocutor. In narratives of personal experience that emerge in formal interviews, interviewer involvement in co-telling often is low (Ochs & Capps 2001). The interviewer generally provides minimum feedback, often restricted to invitations to proceed or to expand on a certain topic and then turns to next issue.

When I met Maria for the first formal interview, I introduced her to an interview practice that would include *low* involvement on my part. "I don't have a structured set of questions to ask," I said. "I want to hear about your break-up, and anything that has to do with it." We were sitting at my office at the shelter and the tape recorder was on. "Let us take your break-up story from the beginning. Maybe you can start by telling me why you left your marriage at this point? I mean, you had lived together for some time and been badly beaten many times. Why did you decide to leave him right now?"

Looking back, I remember that I considered this last question a simple question with the potential to guide Maria into the well-known linear track of telling a narrative with a beginning, middle, and end. I remember that I also considered this way of guiding to be low involvement on my part. I still do in the sense that in relation to what Ochs and Capps referred to, I did not *say* very much and I had indicated that I would remain quite silent during the course of the interview. In retrospect, I realize that I may definitely have formed the plot structure at that moment by imposing a certain temporal order. Thus low or high involvement is not only a question of frequency of words or generally confirming "hmms" or "go ons," it is also about what kind of narrative structure the interviewee guides toward.

However, my attempt to impose a plot structure was not successful. Maria politely rejected my proposal for her narrative beginning. She responded to my question with a short silence and "that is a good question," followed by an "*I really don't know*" and "*I don't think I ever made such a decision*":

> Maria: It was more like . . . that day, a housepainter was doing some work in our living room. I was going to run some errands, so I asked him when he was leaving. "Soon," he said. So I gave him my keys and asked him to lock when he left. I knew my husband was coming home before me, so he could let me in. Once in the street, I was suddenly struck by a feeling of freedom. "I don't have the keys to my home any more," I thought. "I don't have to go back." I just walked around, randomly. All of a sudden, I was standing outside the main police station. I opened the door and went in. "I have something to confess," I said. "The other day I was here with my husband and falsely accused a man of stalking." "I think you should come in and talk to one of our officers," they said. To my surprise they were very friendly. I think I started to cry almost immediately.
>
> You see, a few days earlier, after days and nights of interrogation from my husband, I had accused a totally innocent man, unknown to me, of pursuing me. All the time we lived together, my husband was obsessed with jealousy. He could make up long stories about me and other men, and he went on and on and wanted me to confess things that I had not done with men I did not know. With this man, he believed me. I had done nothing and I didn't know him. But my husband didn't let it end there. He started to go on about him stalking me and made me go to the police with him. It was awful.
>
> After I had made my confession the day I left, they took me to the shelter.

ENDS AND BEGINNINGS

My first impression of Maria's narrative was that it was totally relational—all what she was talking about included good, well-meaning people. It was open in time, meaning that she put herself in promising, yet vulnerable positions in these relations. In subsequent readings I found that she consistently was sideshadowing the present time in her story. By "shadowing the present from the side" the events that happened that day lose some temporal legitimacy and cannot be regarded exclusively as the only possible version of what happened. What she narrated as the actual events in that present moment were, instead, moved into a universe where there were *many* potential presents lying in wait for an opportunity to be triggered into action. What might have happened if the housepainter had said "No, I don't want to have responsibility for your keys," or if Maria had not been struck by a sense of freedom when she had left her keys with him? When she was walking around randomly, what would have happened if she had met someone who asked what she was doing? What would have happened if the police had treated her as a criminal rather than as a victim when she came and confessed that she had accused an innocent man falsely? All these possibilities were present in Maria's narrative, but they were never made explicit. They produced a sense of uncertainty in the narrative, a sense of her not being in control of the situation. "Sideshadows conjure the ghostly presence of might-have-beens or might-bes," Morson writes, "While we see what did happen, we also see the image of what else could have happened. In this way, the hypothetical shows through the actual and so achieves its own shadowy existence in the text" (Morson, 1994, p. 118).

What would have happened if Maria had used the same sideshadowing techniques that had moved her narrative in a more optimistic direction when it came to what the possibilities could mean? What if she had altered the present in her narrative and started off by talking about how isolated, fearful and full of low expectations she had been when she met a housepainter who brought some light into her run-down living room, an activity that foreboded a brighter life, but in another room? Maria would probably have left anyway sooner or later, but she and I might never have met because she might not have had the same need to close time, trying to secure a bright future. Perhaps "bright futures" in her understanding of them were related to open time? All hypothetical but possible plots for other kinds of break-ups and break-up stories.

What also struck me was that at the day of her break-up, Maria reached out to other people but never asked for help. She did not go to the police for seeking help or to report, but to confess. From what she told me later, I learned that guilt feelings were a major issue in her life. Throughout her life, she had been tormented by feelings of insufficiency, and particularly in relation to her husband: When he started to accuse her of not loving him enough or of being interested in other men, she did all she could to convince him that he was wrong. When he first brought the subject up they were not married—so she proposed to him to convince him. However, in the long run she was helpless. To confess that her helplessness and insufficiency had been so extensive as to involve a total stranger was a relief.

It is possible to play around with time while reading Maria's narrative. It could be read as a narrative of how her "old" life and marriage ended, but it could also be read as a narrative of the first day in her "new" life— or as a middle part of something that could be called a "bridge-building" break-up narrative, embracing the "old" as well as the "new." Whether it is the one or the other is not something that can be decided once and for all. It depends on the wider context in which it is told and can fill many different purposes and thereby also be "recycled" many times.

NARRATIVES OF VIOLENCE
SHADOWED BY VORTEX TIME

Violence was not an issue in Maria's family of origin. She had never feared being beaten. She had not experienced much of male dominance and female subordination, more the opposite. She described her father as "a kind and compliant man" and her mother as the "controlling party." In the beginning of their relationship, Maria and her husband lived along egalitarian lines. They shared everything, including their interest in art and literature. Later on their relationship was more characterized by complementarities. He was unemployed from time to time and she was the sole breadwinner. That was all right with her, but not with him. When the first blow hit her, she was totally unprepared. It was in connection with accusations that she had been looking at another man:

> Maria: I had never experienced violence before I met him, so when he slapped me for the first time, I just couldn't believe it. I just didn't let it sink in. I got a black eye, but I didn't let it mean anything to me. I think I just forgot all about it.

I remember that Maria's short narrative filled me with horror. It seemed to me that in all its littleness it was an almost perfect narrative of how a crisis can be produced. She reported a long sequence of escalating disasters: He slapped her, she got a black eye, she did not believe it, she did not let it sink in and she did not let it mean anything to her and *just forgot all about it*. It made her previous narrative of "the last day of my old life and the first day of my new life" even stronger: Was she not happy to have been able to get out? It could have ended very, very badly.

I think what is exposed in Maria's second narrative is a radically different temporal form compared with the sideshadowing of the first. Morson (1994) calls it *vortex time:*

> Vortex time and sideshadowing work in opposite ways. If in sideshadowing apparently simple events ramify into multiple futures, in vortex time an apparent diversity of causes all converge on a single catastrophe. A hidden clock seems to synchronize this diversity so that, even though causal lines seem unrelated to one another, they not only lead to the same result but also do so at the same moment. (p. 163)

Vortex time forebodes disaster. Placed as the beginning or the middle, narratives of violence shadowed by vortex time forebode total destruction as the end of the break-up narrative. So when Maria told me that she gradually woke up from her trance, I was relieved. She said she began to perceive his violence as something that he "just did." When it seemed to her that he more and more avoided letting what he was doing "sink in" and showed no remorse, she tried to take control. It soon became a full-time assignment:

> **Maria:** He totally absorbed me. I had to check on him all the time, you know. It was like "what was he up to, in what mood was he, what was he saying, could I do this, could I do that—no, I better don't, he might be angry with me." These questions were constantly within me. I couldn't do anything without thinking about whether it would suit him or not. I did all this because I wanted to avoid trouble. I couldn't avoid it, but I could reduce it.

Although I concluded that her life had taken a tragic turn, I was pleased to find this narrative, foreshadowing a life without violence. I found it tragic, because her life at that time seemed totally preoccupied with her efforts to escape violence. I found it encouraging for the same reason: She was devoted to the task of securing herself. I read her narrative as one where previous struggles for alternative events were doomed and deluded. Security was the premium task and she would take the steps she had to take to achieve it.

THE USE OF MULTIPLE TEMPORALITIES

Maria's way of using different temporal frameworks within the same narrative and thereby giving a sense of movement and insecurity to the break-up narrative was a basic structure that was repeated in the other women's narratives. By casting shadows over the present from the side, time was opened up for possibilities of ways of ending the violence, endings foreshadowing a life without violence and closing time in a favorable way. Sometimes these sideshadows endow the break-up narrative with a sense of presence of the positive, unexpected and mysterious—sometimes the possibilities are of a negative kind. The presence of negative possibilities is emphasized when vortex time is used in some parts of the break-up narrative. As an example, I will present Eva, a young woman of 26 and the mother of two young children. Listening to her often filled me with the feeling that she had escaped the threat of a disaster by very little:

> **Eva:** I was so young when I met him (her first abusive husband). I mean, I have never had a normal relationship, if you see what I mean. It was more like "if you get beaten, you get beaten"; it's not the end of the world. I think I have developed the wrong way of thinking. I mean, I know it is wrong to beat each other or to assault someone, that's not it, but I haven't lived with a man in any other

way. So I think one starts to categorize the hitting, like a box on the ear is *nothing* . . . then, when they start to handle you real roughly, like kicking and banging your head into the wall, I think that's really awful.

Do you see what I mean? I have categorized it, kind of. Every time I have been beaten up, it doesn't matter how serious, I have thought "I'll wait 'til next time, when it's worse."

It was not like it was acceptable, none of it. It was more like some events were less bad, some were worse. I kind of excused myself with "I don't have enough proof to report him to the police."

Eva moved away from home at an early age. She has lived in two relationships, both with very violent men from the West Indies. When she was beaten by the first husband it was unexpected, but violence was not unknown to her. She had been beaten by her father when she was little. Her mother had been unable to protect her and had denied knowing that she had been beaten, although Eva was sure she knew. Soon after her first husband's first blow, violence was part of her life. In her second relationship with an abusive man, she handled it by categorizing it: It could be bad, worse, and the worst. When it got to be the "worst" she would report it to the police.

When I listened to her, and she started to list increasingly serious violence—a box on the ear, kicking, banging her head into the wall—an inevitable catastrophe seemed to becoming closer and closer. When this line was accompanied by utterance such as "I have never had a normal relationship" and "it was more like if you get beaten, you get beaten, it's not the end of the world," the road to destruction seemed to lie there as straight as an arrow ahead of her. The line of disastrous events was slightly interspersed with remarks about resistance she put up along the way, remarks such as "I know it is wrong to beat each other or assault someone," or "it was not like it was acceptable, none of it." Such utterances cast a somewhat bleak foreshadow from a nonviolent future, unfortunately cut off by remarks such as "I'll wait 'til next time, when it's worse, to report him to the police." What if there is no next time, because he kills you?

I could get quite desperate with her way of presenting her life with two violent men. "You endured too much," I thought. "You are young and therefore careless about your life. You are not frightened enough to protect yourself." When she used more sideshadowing techniques, I found some openings and became a little more optimistic: "You know it is wrong and you have resisted the violence for so long. Use that power to benefit in yours and your children's favor."

Eva's narrative, it seemed to me, was full of questions, not about *if* the violence would come to an end, but about *when* and by *whom* it was to be ended. When "the worst" had happened, or more randomly? By her leaving him or when the catastrophe happened and he had killed her?

The questions of *when* and by *whom* were rendered through the break-up narrative, in which plot and questions were interwoven in complex ways. They seemed to operate in two different social spaces and exist in parallel. In one space, acts of resistance could be performed, acts that were sideshadowed in the narrative, thereby suggesting that every moment involves a whole field of possibilities. In another space, acts of endurance could be performed, acts that were described in vortex time in the narrative, thereby suggesting that the struggle for alternatives was doomed. Nonacceptance of the violence was the combining link between the two. Eva told me this:

> Eva: I have been more like a dog. When they (the men) were a little bit nice, I felt so dammed happy. I mean, what kind of life is that? I just feel, it must come to and end, I don't want to live like this for the rest of my life. Like when I am 35, the kids will be grown up. Then I can live my own life. . . . I have no plans of living as his bloody attribute and becoming bitter.

Eva opens with a tragic statement "I have been more like a dog," a statement that could be viewed as the utmost sign of endurance. However, expressions of nonacceptance run through her account—"I don't want to live like this for the rest of my life, what kind of a life is that, etc.," as do expressions of resistance, "I just feel, it must come to an end." Both ways of accounting, I would argue, forebode the break-up and may therefore be understood as the beginning of the break-up story. The beginning is then followed by a middle, where the two narrative themes, endurance and resistance, form the main plot along parallel or more interwoven lines.

Expressions of resistance were not always easy to identify in break-up narratives. Whereas usually it is possible to look for obvious signs of resistance in these cases, it is necessary to search for clues of "small" acts with resisting power, acts that may include ways of avoiding him, "double-play strategies" with compliance on the surface and rebellion underneath. The "rebellion underneath" included plans of breaking up. The narratives contained fewer examples of overt resistance. Endurance was omnipresent but not valued as an appreciated capacity.

MAKING MORAL JUDGMENTS: THE TRANSFORMATION OF PAST INTO PRESENT

Some parts of Eva's break-up story included backshadowing of her behavior during her last marriage. She was very dissatisfied with herself. Her dissatisfaction could be worded as *I should have behaved differently:*

> Eva: I think it is so embarrassing, I'm so ashamed. It doesn't matter if
> everyone says I shouldn't be, I'm ashamed anyway, 'cause I was
> so d . . . d stupid to let myself be treated like that.
> Margareta: When you say you're so embarrassed when you think about
> what you let happen, what comes to mind?
> Eva: I mean things like, why I let him hit me and terrorize me in the first
> place, it's really more my style to say: OK this is the end of it
> Margareta: What do you mean let yourself?
> Eva: That's because today I'd have . . . he hit me a whole lot you know.
> I must have been an idiot to let it go on. Why didn't I report him
> to the police the very first time he punched me?
> Margareta: Is that what you mean by "admitting" that you didn't
> report him to the police?
> Eva: Yes.
> Margareta: Because I assume that you didn't think it really was OK for
> this to happen?
> Eva: No, no I definitely don't think it is OK but I mean that the way I
> acted showed that I allowed it indirectly. By not calling the police,
> I acted as if I accepted him hitting me and treating me like shit.

In this exchange, my involvement is quite high. What I am doing is basically to oppose "Eva-now" when she attacks the "Eva-back-then." "One key problem with backshadowing lies in its assumption that the past contained legible signs of the future. Were such signs in fact present and visible? Were there not also countless other possibilities?" Morson (1994, p. 234) asks. "Of course, there were," I would answer. "Of course there were, and of course Eva knew it." Why did she exclude all the other possibilities in her narrative?

In a positive way, I think the exclusion of all other possibilities expresses superiority and excellence. Eva is very satisfied with what she has accomplished. Her previous narratives strengthen the impression that she has done something extraordinary by leaving this very violent man. With such power and competence, why didn't she do it long ago? Her satisfaction also includes resistance and anger which, in the social space of her marriage, was not possible to discharge. In a not very positive way, I think the exclusion of all other possibilities expresses contempt for different kinds of weaknesses—including not having been able to eliminate all sideshadows and including not having the power to look into the future. Such contempt produces a breeding ground for self-hatred and poor self-confidence.

CONCLUDING REMARKS

My opening argument was that breaking up is about difference and movement and contained the power for identity (re)formation. The break-up narrative plays in important role in determining along which lines the (re)formed life history can be developed, I added to that argument.

The most obvious difference is the most fundamental one, I will conclude—that of the difference in social space made by leaving an abusive husband. When the woman leaves him, she leaves the violent marriage, a social space basically organized in his interest. She enters into various kinds of spaces of "the Other." One of the first steps in that journey made by the women whose stories I shared was that of seeking shelter at a refuge for battered women. This dislocation of the marital space and relocation to the space of the Other, was of fundamental importance to the break-up narrative. In part, this difference *was* the narrative. Without this relocation the women's narratives would have been so constrained by situational conditions that they might never even have existed. Simply speaking, in the space of a marriage organized in the abusive man's interest there are no tellers and listeners to battered women's break-up stories.

The second difference—that of difference in time—was just as fundamental. When I started to listen to what the women had to tell, I had the idea that the break-up stories would be structured along the traditional lines, in which loose ends are eliminated and a beginning, middle, and end are created—all leading to the privileging of the narrative moment when the entire narrative pattern is purportedly visible. This never happened. As a result, in the break-up narratives the women shared with me, the past does not look as if it were predestined to lead to the present. The past may be omnipresent or it may be backshadowed by the present. The future may be the constituting factor and foreshadow the present; the end may be the beginning and the beginning the end. My conclusion is, however, that the women and I had the idea—the aspiration even—to construct neat narratives structured by linear time with all loose ends nicely tied up. We all paid a price for that aspiration.

I paid the smallest price in that I had to leave my ingrained opinions about narrative structure, slightly reorganize my interviews, and become more attentive to the women's way of structuring their stories. Maria paid a higher price in that she insisted on foreshadowing her life, thereby eliminating loose ends that might have been valuable to explore further. Eva paid the highest price in that she insisted in backshadowing her behavior in her marriage and started accusing herself. What can be learned from this is the importance of giving support and acceptance to narrators who uses different temporal frameworks when trying to make a whole of the experiences that constitute their respective break-up processes. This sense, I am sure, requires an outsider, a person who listens from an external standpoint. I think Maria was right when she encouraged the other women at the shelter to share their stories and then took me on board as their external listener—most often with a low involvement but sometimes with higher involvement when I wanted to explore, question, and oppose.

168   *Margareta Hydén*

ACKNOWLEDGMENT

The study was supported by a grant from The Swedish Research Council.

REFERENCES

Hydén, M. (1994). *Woman battering as marital act*. Oslo: Scandinavian University Press.
Hydén, M. (1999). The world of the fearful: Battered women's narratives of leaving abusive husbands. *Feminism & Psychology, 9*, 449–469.
Hydén, M. (2005) "I must have been an idiot to let it go on": Agency and positioning in battered women's narratives of leaving. *Feminism & Psychology, 15*, 171–190.
Hydén, M. (2008). Narrating sensitive topics. In M. Andrews, C. Squire, & M. Tamboukou (Eds.), *Doing narrative research*. London: Sage.
Hydén, M., & McCarthy, I. (1994). Woman battering and father-daughter incest disclosure: Discourses of denial and acknowledgement. *Discourse & Society, 5*, 543–565.
Labov, W. (2006). Narrative pre-construction. *Narrative Inquiry, 16*, 37–45.
Morson, G. S. (1994). *Narrative and freedom. The shadows of time*. New Haven, CT: Yale University Press.
Ochs, E., & Capps, L. (2001). *Living narrative. Creating lives in everyday storytelling*. Cambridge, MA: Harvard University Press.

10 Beyond Narrative
Dementia's Tragic Promise

Mark Freeman

"SOMETIMES YOU JUST LIVE TOO LONG"

I shall begin this essay by referring briefly to two conversations I recently had with my mother, who suffers from dementia. In the first, she was complaining, yet again, about her living situation. Just over a year earlier, she had moved into an assisted living residence. She had done so reluctantly but (more or less) willingly: Given some of the difficulties she had been having with cooking, cleaning, and other such activities, and given as well the occasional loneliness of living by herself, she had come to see that she might be better off elsewhere. But this has brought difficulties of its own, not the least of which concerns the fact that most of the time she has no idea at all why she is there and resents it immensely. A new woman just moved in, she told me last week. And apparently, every time she's finished with dinner she asks my mother where the Bingo game is being played. "She asks the same question over and over again!," my mother complained angrily. "She's stupid!" "It's got nothing to do with stupidity," I tell her; "it sounds like she's got some memory problems, and if truth be known (I add, as gently as possible), they're similar to yours." My mother is momentarily speechless, both knowing and not-knowing at the same time. And then a couple of minutes later she tells the same story once more, displaying through her own repetition the exact same malady she has just condemned.

I, too, am speechless.

The other conversation was quite different. My mother had left me a panicky telephone message about people coming to visit her, but she was confused about the details and needed to speak with me. "I think Lissy (her daughter-in-law) is picking me up tonight to take me to the Cape," she said. I told her I seriously doubted that; having spoken to Lissy just the night before, I knew that she had plans to take my mother to the Cape 2 weeks later. A day earlier, she had been convinced that her sister was coming to visit the following day and that my brother, Ken, and his wife were visiting a week from then. "No," I had told her, "I am quite sure Ken is coming to your place tomorrow." Did that mean that she was having multiple visitors tomorrow? "Call your sister," I said, "and see when she's coming, this week or next; and then, call me so I know who's coming when." Her sister was in fact coming the following week. So, Ken was visiting tomorrow, her sister next week. Fine. But just after things had settled down, she had received the call from Lissy. This was what led to her coming undone. It was information overload; everything was getting jumbled together; the visitors were the same and the dates of visit were the same but they had become severed from one another. And so, when she woke up the next morning, and tried to piece together this awful, confusing puzzle, panic set in. At this point I simply tried to calm her down and reassure her that only one person, Ken, was coming to visit this weekend. Her sister was coming the following weekend, and Lissy, the one after that. Just to make sure, I told her I would call Lissy. Yes, she was planning to visit in 2 weeks. So I called my mother back right away to confirm the situation. It was at that moment that she broke down, bewildered, over the very being she had become. "Oh, Mark, *what am I going to do?* Sometimes you just live too long. . . . "

"I WANT TO BE A PERSON"

My mother currently exists in a kind of liminal psychic space. Despite her occasional recognition of her difficulties, as above, she either downplays them (She's actually spoken lightheartedly of having "CRS" [Can't Remember Shit] syndrome) or is (virtually) unaware of them. She also remains vehement about her abilities. "I know I can still drive just fine," she will say. "I've always taken care of my own papers." "I've never been late with a check." If I question these abilities—"Ma, there's a chance you'll get lost when you're driving." "Your papers are in a state of chaos." "Actually, you *have* been late with several checks"—her response is often swift and to the point: "You're treating me like a child." Or: "I'm not an imbecile." I sometimes find myself trying to explain to her that things are different now, that some of the things she used to be able to do, very competently, she can no longer do. "I want to get some kind of job," she announced recently, maybe office work of the sort she had done years ago. "That really may not be the best job for you at this point," I told her. "There are some things you can do just fine," I said, "but other things are harder for you now." Generally speaking, however, it doesn't sink in. It is difficult to determine whether this is a function of incomprehension or denial or both.

As nice as it is, the assisted-living residence where she has landed undoubtedly adds to the problem. "Bus trips to get ice cream!" "Bingo, every night!" "Everybody goes upstairs to bed at 8 o'clock!" Many of her peers have walkers or wheelchairs and look very old and fragile. She doesn't look like them at all; she's attractive and moves briskly, still confident in her step. Consequently, these people, and the activities they pursue, annoy and sometimes upset her. We therefore find ourselves looking for ways to help her, unsure whether "adjustment" is the answer or something else entirely.

"What do you want?," I asked her recently. The answer: "*I want to be a person.*" When she had lived alone, she said, she had been a "free agent," able to walk over to the local drugstore, to come and go as she pleased. And she could drive. Now, however, there was that rickety old van. And there were all those old people. To paraphrase her: It's all just nothingness.

There is an image still in view, of a full and whole person: independent, free, of sound mind and body. There is a story that can be told about this person. It is the story of a child whose parents were too poor to keep her and who therefore sent her off to a children's home—which she had quite loved— for a couple of years. It is the story of a teenager, a bit shy but the smartest in the whole class; of a young woman, competent and hardworking, going it alone, while her husband was away in India during the war; of a middle-aged woman, prematurely widowed, who, after years of being a homemaker, had to go out into the work world once more, where she excelled, rising to the position of office manager, in charge of lots of people and able to make the whole outfit run smoothly and efficiently. This story still seems to be with her. How dare anyone suggest that she could no longer balance a checkbook! She had balanced books for a living, and was damn good at it! On one level, the continued presence of this story is surely a good thing. But it is also the source of much of her current frustration and sorrow.

For better and for worse, she simply *forgets* many of the things she has been unable to do; she has minimal memory of her lost purse or checkbook (or whatever) and, if we apprise her of these losses, she generally seems not to believe it. Not unlike many others with dementia, what she often does, in fact, is convince herself that these things must have been taken from her, perhaps stolen. It cannot possibly be me, she is in effect telling us; it has to be someone else—maybe one of the workers in her residence. She believes this despite the fact that we have managed to locate, eventually, every single item she has lost. The same is true of plans we might make together. Recently, for instance, I asked her whether she wanted to spend some time with my brother Ken, whom I introduced earlier, and his family. It would be a change of scenery. Plus, her great-granddaughter would be there. "Sure," she said. "That sounds wonderful." We even spoke about what weekend she might go. But she forgot all of this. And when she (re)learned that she would soon be leaving to visit my brother and his family, she immediately became convinced that we had orchestrated the entire thing behind her back, as usual, treating her like a child once again. And there was, there is, nothing one can do to convince her of the truth. For the most part, we no longer even try.

There are also times when she "remembers" things that didn't happen. Just recently, in the wake of yet another misplaced purse, she told me she had left it at my house when she had been over for dinner. This simply wasn't true. But in her mind it was, and remains so; and as a result, my wife and I become magically transformed into the purse snatchers: It's *our* fault that she doesn't have that purse, and we really ought to take the time to find it. Here, too, there is absolutely nothing that can be done to move her from her convictions: On the whole, her ego remains strong and resilient enough to utterly reject the reality before her.

Herein lies her liminal status. Much of the time, she is—subjectively— who she has always been: an office manager and checkbook balancer, able to do just fine, thank you, on her own. ("So, buzz off with all your 'help!'") This identity is sometimes profoundly interrupted, however, and, much to her horror, the story she has been able to tell herself suddenly comes undone. At these times, she is living a broken narrative. And it is made all the more painful by the felt permanence of the break: There will be no fixing it; the disease is marching forward, inexorably; she is hurtling toward the end. She is having more of these kinds of desperate moments. But she often forgets having had them. So she's still looking toward the future, the new apartment, the new job, the new *life* that will allow her to recover what's been taken away. Desperate moments are thus replaced by ones that are a curious amalgam of frustration, rage, and hope.

There are other kinds of moments as well, however, and they are telling ones. My mother has always loved music, especially when it's played outdoors on a nice summer day. And so, this past summer my wife and I took her to as many concerts as we possibly could. She's utterly engaged when she's there: totally connected to the music, moving to it, usually like no one else around. Top it off with a glass or two of wine and some good food and she's where she wants to be. There are few moments in her life when she is happier, more at peace. Apparently, the story was much the same when she spent those few days with her great-granddaughter. Pushing the baby in her stroller, up and down a clean suburban street, she had been freed, if only temporarily, of her burdens. She has become divested of self, of ego. There is neither a broken narrative nor the stubbornly continuous one that provides so much fuel for her frustration. There is just music, just Sophie. Life becomes worthwhile again.

Life therefore becomes most worthwhile for her precisely when *she*— qua autobiographical identity—isn't there. Or, to put the matter somewhat differently, if paradoxically, her healthiest and most life-affirming experiences as a self, a vital self, are precisely when her autobiographical identity, and narrative, are in abeyance. There does remain a self in these instances: the self who loves music (and always has), the self who loves Sophie (and always will). But it is a self that is rooted mainly in the present, in the living moment, in the relation to what is *Other*. Her identity at these moments, therefore, is not so much a *narrative* identity, born out of the particulars of her history, as what might be considered a kind of ontological or spiritual identity, born out of her being, out of those less particularized dimensions of history that become sedimented in the form of our interests, inclinations, and passions. These are moments of *being present* and indeed being-*in*-the-present, and the very energy and vitality they are able to generate may well tell us something about the limits, even the dangers, of narrative.

Music and great-grandchildren, among other things, provide an occasion for what Iris Murdoch has referred to as "unselfing," a process wherein the otherness of the Other displaces ego concerns. "We cease to be," she writes, "in order to attend to the existence of something else, a natural object, a person in need" (1970, p. 58). Here is another passage that nicely spells out Murdoch's perspective:

> I am looking out of my window in an anxious and resentful state of mind, oblivious of my surroundings, brooding perhaps on some damage done to my prestige. Then suddenly I observe a hovering kestrel. In a moment everything is altered. The brooding self with its hurt vanity has disappeared. There is nothing now but kestrel. And when I return to thinking of the other matter it seems less important. (p. 82)

The *world* has returned, and it has done so at precisely the same moment that the (autobiographical) self and its narrative have "disappeared." What are the implications of this unselfing process about which Murdoch speaks?

BEYOND NARRATIVE

This process would seem to lead us beyond narrative, if not for the whole of our existence then at least for a significant portion of it. I am reminded in this context of Crispin Sartwell's recent book *End of Story* (2000), which is essentially a diatribe against narrative. Much of our experience, Sartwell reminds us, escapes linguistic articulation. It therefore strikes him as ironic, and wrong, that so much attention has come to be devoted to narrative as a lens for understanding the human world. In addition, however, there is the idea that narrative, in its fetish for organization, order, *coherence,* is an oppressive force that we would do well to move beyond. Sartwell even offers a kind of confession early on in the book:

> I've tried to live my own life with an extreme degree of coherence; I've tried to understand my own life as a techne, to dedicate it to the realization of well-defined goals. I've tried to rationalize my life: both to live it rationally and to convince myself that I have lived or am living it rationally. I reached a point at which I came to experience the need to do that as a torture. I came to experience the recalcitrance of myself to my will, came to experience the immensity of my own horrible and lovely irrationality. I came also to experience or to admit the recalcitrance of the world to my will. The latter recalcitrance I could initially narrate as a series of "barriers" to my life-plan. But I reached the point at which I wanted to learn to let the world be instead of trying to transform it into an instrument of my will. (pp. 15–16)

This "torture," and the liberation that followed as Sartwell sought to move beyond narrative in his own life, apparently provided him with a lesson about the underside of narrative itself: It can become a kind of prison that reduces the bountifulness of experience and subjects it to willful control. There is thus the need for "letting go," for disordering one's world; only then will the "ecstasy" of experience be made possible: "The moment of ecstasy is a moment of vertigo, a vertigo that responds to letting go of one's projects into an all-encompassing present moment" (p. 22).

As Sartwell goes on to argue, drawing especially on Bataille's *Inner Experience* (1988), itself a kind of diatribe against "project," against "the putting off of existence to a later point" by virtue of one's recourse to "discursive thought" (p. 46), narrative is undermined, deconstructed, by the sheer force of certain modes of experience: "Narrative comes apart at the extremes . . . in ecstasy, in writhing pain, at death" (Sartwell, 2000, p. 65). But that is not all: "[Narrative] has already also come apart everywhere, all the time, wherever people are breathing, or walking around, or watching TV, and not getting anywhere narratively speaking. What narrative is inadequate to is not just the shattering moment, but the moment of indifference" (p. 65). Sartwell even offers us some instruction in this context:

> You cannot narrate if you cannot breathe, so shut up for a moment and take a deep breath. Pull yourself away from significance for a moment and let yourself feel the sweet, deep, all-enveloping insignificance all around you. And take comfort in your own insignificance; take comfort in the triviality of your culture; take comfort in the triviality of your life-project and your failure in realizing. (p. 65)

Take comfort in the fact that, even though you can't drive, or get a job, or maintain your own books, and that consequently you're no longer a Person, you're still alive, well-fed and well-clothed, able to find meaning in music or joy in your great-grandchild. Sartwell's message is ultimately a quite simple one: *Just chill.* Forget about all that "significance" stuff; indifference will undoubtedly leave you a good deal more content with your lot in life. I have been tempted to think in similar terms to Sartwell myself: *Get over it;* get over your*self,* with your still-kicking projects, your aspirations and fantasies. But this is precisely what my mother cannot do. She's in too deep.

Sartwell can surely identify with this problem. He speaks of feeling the need for meaning as a "pressure, as an anxiety, and furthermore as the project of having some project, and hence as a project that can never be discharged. I live like this," he admits: "busy trying to finish whatever's in front of me as quickly as possible. Then finished. Then feeling empty, subject to attack from my own head. Then inventing or accepting a new project. And so on. I work by projects toward the extinction of project, then can't live there and go on to a new one" (p. 65). So it is that he must tell himself: *Just chill.* But it's hard: Whether we're narrativists or antinarrativists, the pressure for meaning, for significance, remains much the same. All he can do, therefore, is try to find some relief. As he does: in caring for his children (who he's "not trying to make . . . into particular sorts of people"), in playing the accordion or the harmonica (neither of which he's trying to "master"). "OK," he avows; playing these instruments is "still trying to do something." So perhaps there's a narrative in there somewhere (the college professor who, much to his chagrin, gets so caught up in trying to defeat discursive thought through discursive thought that he's got to find devices that provide some measure of "surcease from the voice in my head"). "But the point is that the purpose is achieved precisely at the moment that it fades from awareness, those moments are the extinction of project sought by project" (p. 65). He wishes he "could live there more, that [he] could play more," that there could be "deeper and longer forms of immersion" (p. 66). I wish this for my mother, too. In her case, however, it would seem that there is only one thing that could make this wish come true: the very dissolution of her own autobiographical identity—which, of course, will only happen if and when her dementia has run its destructive course. Shall we wish for *this*? It would indeed likely provide her some "surcease" of her own. At the same time, she will also have moved that much closer to oblivion (indifference?) and death. What a strange situation. Is there anything to do now, in the face of her more liminal state of being?

DECONSTRUCTING THE CULTURAL STORY

I have some misgivings about Sartwell's rendition of narrative: Narrative need not be as coercive and controlling as he sometimes suggests, and, whether we like it or not, it surely remains intimately connected to what we generally think of as selfhood. (Perhaps this is why Sartwell's own account of how he has tried to move beyond narrative itself takes the form of a narrative.) My mother's recent experience, however, has allowed me to see his argument in a somewhat different light. It is quite possible that by moving beyond narrative, beyond the confines of storylines that do indeed serve to oppress her, she too will experience something like liberation.

It is precisely here, at this juncture, that cultural reality becomes particularly salient. For, in the background of so much of my mother's frustration and discontent is, as suggested earlier, a highly robust image of who and what she ought to be—manifested in the form of an equally robust, if deluded, image of who she actually is now. Perhaps this is a universal phenomenon. Perhaps, that is, human beings, wherever we may find them, reject quite naturally their cognitive decline and spontaneously devise strategies for convincing themselves and others it's not happening. It is also possible, however, that a portion of my mother's response to her current situation is the product of a culture that, in a distinct sense, refuses to admit the reality of decline, and death, into its midst. "Stop Aging Now!" is a phrase that one sometimes sees in conjunction with plastic surgery and skin creams designed to remove all traces of time, all the wear and tear of growing old.

There is a dual cultural narrative at work in this context, therefore, operating behind the scenes of consciousness. There is the narrative of the vital, self-sufficient Individual, who resists the kind of fragility, vulnerability, and dependency that growing old sometimes brings in tow. It has come as something of a surprise to see just how potent this narrative is in my mother's case. It is highly resistant to modification too: As of now, there remains little room for building in a sense of fragility or vulnerability, little room for admitting that things are changing. In part, this is no doubt because of the unconscious dimension of the narrative at hand. It is not something she can look at, hold at a distance. Rather, it is working through her, permeating her being. In some earlier work (Freeman, 2002, 2006), I have spoken in this context of the "narrative unconscious," which has to do with those parts of our *history* that have not, or not yet, become an explicit part of our *story*.

There is an added feature of the narrative of self-sufficiency as well, one that seems extremely potent in American culture in particular. In the present case, it has to do with my mother's fervent wish not to be a "burden" on anyone—especially, of course, her children. One of the reasons being unable to drive is so frustrating to her is that others—most often, my wife or me—have to do it for her. "I hate to rely so much on you," she often says. "I hate to be a burden." "It's not a big deal," we may say in response. "It's just part of life." But it's not part of the life—part of the narrative of life—that she has employed throughout the years. I have even tried to deconstruct this narrative with her: "People can rely upon one another," I might say; our lives are intertwined; we're not monads but relational beings, and it really is okay that we're doing this with you and for you. "Thank you, thank you, thank you," she sometimes says when we return her home. She is extremely appreciative for the "buggy ride," as she calls it. But she very much wishes she didn't have to take it. The narrative of self-sufficiency looms large for her.

This narrative is reinforced by another, with which it operates in tandem: the narrative of inexorable decline—which may culminate in "narrative foreclosure," as I have called it, wherein one becomes convinced that "the story's over" (Freeman, 2000). Old people, with their walkers and their wheelchairs, surround my mother. People sit in the lobby, slumped over, dozing, waking briefly when there are passersby. Some of them do seem to have little to do, little left to live for: Their story *is* over—or at least that is how they see it. And part of the reason *why* they see it this way may be linked back to the image of that vital self just considered. They are the inverted image of that self, beyond vitality, beyond self-sufficiency—in some ways, my mother has suggested, beyond personhood itself.

She is vehemently *not*-them. The nightly Bingo that they play downstairs, in open view, really gets to her. At the end of the day, there are only mindless games, camaraderie created by random numbers. Time for them is not to be lived, but passed. There is no story to be told after such days; they are just like the one before and the one before that. My mother sometimes seems to resent these "nonpersons" with their nonstories. In her eyes, they have crossed the line, and the image of them sitting there, night after night, is painful to behold. I suppose one could say that, on some level, they exist in the moment. And it's quite possible that they are less troubled by their existence than she is hers. But this is hardly an occasion for envy.

DILEMMAS OF BEING

As of now, she is simply not ready to go there. That is, she is not ready to join the ranks of these seeming nonpersons and, painful though it is, is thus holding fast to what remains of her own personhood, her own autobiographical identity. She still wants to live a life that is worth telling about, one in which meaningful and significant things happen, and can be communicated to other people. This brings about problems of its own. Sometimes, a trip will be planned—a river cruise, to take one recent example. The hope is that the trip will serve as an Event—that is, a meaningful and significant enough episode to be recounted, gratefully. "How was the trip, ma?" We nervously await her answer. Sometimes, her face is filled with excitement and she eagerly tells the story of the day. But more often, it proves to be disappointing. "We just sat in a boat. We really didn't *do* anything." And the picture can become darker still due to the fact that she may not remember much about the trip at all. She often complains about there being a lack of activities where she lives. She's right; there ought to be more. We have come to realize, however, that many of the activities that do take place—and which she apparently participates in—are quickly forgotten, thereby leading her, again and again, to the conclusion that there is simply nothing to do there. "But ma," we might say, "you *do* do things there." Materially speaking, this is true. Psychically speaking, however, it is false. And it's her psyche that is leading the way.

In a distinct sense, we become the selves we fashion through the imagination. My mother has thus become the self that she has imagined through the events, the nonevents, and the forgotten events of her life. She complained recently about feeling like "nothing." This is no doubt because there is so much "nothing" in the past that she daily looks back upon when we ask her what she did and how it went. (It is getting close to the time for us to stop asking these kinds of questions.) She often can't remember what went on in a given day and, as noted before, concludes that there has been nothing at all. Or there are hazy scenes, built up out of memories and fantasies, today's images and yesterday's and maybe tomorrow's. This hazy nothingness is what there is, and it doesn't resolve itself very well in the form of a story worth telling. Nor does it lead to the kind of self she remembers having been and still wants to be.

Some of what I am describing here is likely a function of the biological process of memory loss as it is found in dementia. Short-term memory declines before long-term, and as a result personal identity is less rooted in the near than in the distant past. This brings us closer to the heart of the existential problem at hand: There remain memories of the vital, self-sufficient self my mother once was. Indeed, those memories remain compelling enough to enter the present: In her own mind, there's a significant part of her that *is* that self, still. At the same time, however, this vision of the self cannot be confirmed and sustained by the day-to-day reality she lives. For, that reality, bound up as it is with the passing events of the day, is much more transient, much more evanescent. It seems that there is nothing to get hold of. Or, to put it just a bit differently, all that can be gotten hold of is: nothing. It's the juxtaposition of these two realities, tied to the distant and the near past, the self that was and the self that is, that makes things so difficult.

There are three dilemmas—let us call them "dilemmas of being"—I want to refer to in summing up the present situation. On the one hand, my mother is tired and frustrated, feeling at times that her life has gone on long enough. She has no interest in spiraling downhill, descending into madness like some of the people she has known through the years, and wants to avoid it all costs. On the other hand, she remains committed, strenuously, to pressing on, being her own person, keeping herself as connected to the world as possible. This, again, is surely a good thing on some level. But the fact that she has so much difficulty actually *doing* it—that is, conducting her life in the way that she wishes, the way that she once did—makes for a difficult time. She has thus come to be decidedly ambivalent about nothing less than *being* itself. As I have suggested, one of the deep sources of this ambivalence is the culture in which she has lived, with its narratives of self-sufficiency and decline, vitality and loss. She is caught in the middle of these narratives, and at times she cannot help but feel torn about the very substance of her life.

There are times when the admonition to "just chill" is quite appropriate. There are also times when it is possible to deconstruct the cultural story in some small way: Maybe it's okay to be vulnerable, to need people, at least once in a while; maybe the self-sufficiency thing can be taken down a notch. By and large, however, these strategies are not particularly effective. For one, they require a kind of self-consciousness, even a kind of historical consciousness—that is, an awareness of the ways in which cultural narratives have become constitutive of identity—that my mother does not have. (There's just so much I can implore her to engage in deconstructive thinking.) For another, her commitment to the narrative of self-sufficiency, and her dread of the narrative of decline, remain powerful forces in her own ongoing work of being. And work it is: There is hard labor involved in keeping her identity going, challenges every step along the way. We feel an obligation to help her with this labor, to support her in her ontological work. Deconstructive excursions aside, this generally means supporting the narrative of self-sufficiency and helping her maintain her independence to the greatest extent possible—even while recognizing that this very support, this very affirmation of autonomy, may very well have the unintended and undesired consequence of adding to her frustration and anger. "Maybe you *can* get a job," I'll say. "There's nothing preventing you from walking to the store." "There's plenty, still, for you to do in the world." At the same time, of course, I know how difficult all this really is for her. In all likelihood, she is not going to get a job, or walk to the store; and concretely speaking, it is no easy task to determine what she can do, at this juncture in her life, that would be as meaningful and significant as she wants it to be. She simply cannot do some of the things she wishes to do or imagines that she can. And this hurts.

The second dilemma of being brings us back to some of the rather more frightening territory I began to explore earlier. As committed as we may be to affirming my mother's autonomy and helping her retain her sense of independence and efficacy, I confess that there are in fact times when we "look forward" to the future—when a portion of her preoccupation with independence, self-sufficiency, efficacy, *meaning,* will be left behind in the wake of the disease. Needless to say, perhaps, it is very strange to think about this next stage, when she will have essentially left narrative behind. Her arrival at this stage will signify a state of profound loss: In all likelihood, she will no longer know quite who she is—surely not in the sense that she used to know herself, years ago, and probably not in the sense that she knows herself now, in this liminal state I have been discussing. Gone will be that sense of rootedness in a history, in *my* history—my past, my story, my identity as *this* person—that for so long characterizes a "normal" self, at least in the modern West. In a distinct sense, *she* will no longer be here, and we will need to learn to mourn her loss, even while what remains of that earlier person sits at the table, right across from us, moving in and out of familiarity, recognition. My brothers and I dread this future. But she may very well be suffering less, or at least in a different way, than she is now. For, also gone will be that backdrop of expectations and images—and storylines—that right now is causing so much pain.

Will she ultimately be in a "better" place at this point? It is of course difficult to say. It all depends on what remains after narrative, and autobiographical identity, have been left behind. Insofar as she is left with a kind of perpetual nothingness—a state of suspended animation, as it were—it will hardly deserve to be called better, save in the most cursory way. She will have arrived at the land of those "nonpersons" considered earlier: The end of narrative would thus spell the beginning of oblivion, of the very *absence* of Other, of world. And even if it is possible that she would be "just fine," subjectively, her frustration and anger having subsided, rendered essentially irrelevant, it is hard to think of this sort of destination as a better place.

But there is another possibility too, and it has to do with the idea of an ontological or spiritual identity that may continue to exist even after auto-biographical identity has been left behind. In discussing this distinction with a colleague, I was introduced to a similar distinction made by Antonio Damasio in *The Feeling of What Happens* (1999). During the course of development, Damasio suggests, there is a movement from a "core self" to an "autobiographical self." In regard to the former, he writes:

> You know that you are conscious, you feel that you are in the act of know-ing, because the subtle imaged account that is now flowing in the stream of your organism's thoughts exhibits the knowledge that your proto-self has been changed by an object that has just become salient in the mind. You know you exist because the narrative exhibits you as a protagonist in the act of knowing. You rise above the sea level of knowing, transiently but incessantly, as a *felt* core self, renewed again and again, thanks to anything that comes from outside the brain into its sensory machinery or anything that comes from the brain's memory stores toward sensory, motor, or autonomic recall. You know it is *you* seeing because the story depicts a character—you—doing the seeing. (pp. 171–172)

Damasio refers to T.S. Eliot's *Four Quartets* in this context, which speaks of a music "heard so deeply that it is not heard at all," and which states that "you are the music while the music lasts." Eliot, Damasio suggests, was apparently thinking of "the fleeting moment in which a deep knowledge can emerge—a union, or incarnation, as he called it" (p. 172). Damasio's core self thus bears within it a spiritual possibility, connected with the very ineffable nature of "being the music"—or the great-grandchild, the glass of good wine, "anything that comes from outside the brain into its sensory machinery."

It should be noted that, for Damasio, the core self is itself bound up with narrative—albeit of a wordless sort: "Knowing springs to life in the story, it inheres in the newly constructed neural pattern that constitutes the non-verbal account. You hardly notice the storytelling," he avows, "because the images that dominate the mental display are those of the things of which you are now conscious—the objects you see or hear—rather than those that swiftly constitute the feeling of you in the act of knowing" (p. 172). It is difficult to know what to make of this conceptualization: While narrative, or narrativity, may well be a precondition of sorts for achieving the kind of "union" about which Damasio speaks—there remain operative "those less particularized dimensions of history," as I put it earlier, "that become sedi-mented in the form of our interests, inclinations, and passions"—it is not entirely clear that "storytelling" is involved. Be that as it may, this notion of a core self, of a self that is "renewed again and again" through its encounter with the *Other*-than-self, remains an important one.

Now, in the healthy mind, Damasio continues, something does in fact last after the (proverbial) music is gone:

> In complex organisms such as ours, equipped with vast memory capacities, the fleeting moments of knowledge in which we discover our existence are facts that can be committed to memory, be properly categorized, and be related to other memories that pertain both to the past and to the anticipated future. The consequence of that complex learning operation is the development of autobiographical memory, an aggregrate of dispositional records of who we have been physically and of who we have usually been behaviorally, along with records of who we plan to be in the future. We can enlarge this aggregate memory and refashion it as we go through a lifetime. When certain personal records are made explicit in reconstructed images, as needed, in smaller or greater quantities, they become the *autobiographical self.* (pp. 172–173)

Whether Damasio is right to speak of "aggregrates" and "records" is open to question; his terminology bespeaks a kind of substantialism that runs counter to much current thinking about autobiographical memory and the autobiographical self. Nevertheless, the distinction at hand, between the core self and the autobiographical self, is a useful one, in regard to both development and the process of decline as it is observed in dementia and related maladies. In the early stages of development, Damasio suggests, there may be "little more than reiterated states of core self." With continued experience, however, "autobiographical memory grows and the autobiographical self can be deployed" (p. 175). The process of decline, in turn, moves in the reverse direction: "When the loss of memory for past events is marked enough to compromise autobiographical records, the autobiographical self is gradually extinguished and extended consciousness collapses. This happens in advance of the subsequent collapse of core consciousness" (p. 209).

If Damasio is right, the core self remains—for a time—after the demise of the autobiographical self. This brings me to a final dilemma of being, having to do with this idea of the autobiographical self. More and more, I have come to think of this self as a "mixed bag." Some of the reasons have been referred to, both explicitly and implicitly, in this essay. It can bring pride and pleasure, gratification over one's achievements, and much more. But it can also bring regret and disappointment, shame and frustration, particularly when one's self doesn't measure up to cultural and personal expectations and ideals. Following Damasio's line of thinking, the culprit in these situations is none other than the autobiographical self. There is a distinct sense, however, in which the culprit may also be said to be narrative itself. Moving beyond narrative may therefore serve to resolve the dilemmas of being that have been considered herein.

DEMENTIA'S TRAGIC PROMISE

Moving beyond narrative may also clear a space for just that sort of "union" considered earlier. It is a striking fact—and one that is well known to mystics, artists, and many others—that the experiences that move us the most, those sorts of ecstatic or transcendent experiences wherein one feels truly at one with the world, generally entail what Murdoch had referred to as "unselfing," putting aside one's ego and thereby letting in the world, in all of its profound otherness. I have come to speak in this context of "the priority of the Other," seeing in mysticism especially a profound and important challenge to the legacy of the self (see Freeman, 2004).

Murdoch's preferred vehicle of unselfing is great art, which "teaches us how real things can be looked at and loved without being seized and used, without being appropriated into the greedy organism of the self. This exercise of *detachment*," as Murdoch calls it (somewhat problematically, I think; she seems to be considering a process rather more relational), "is difficult and valuable whether the thing contemplated is a human being or the root of a tree or the vibration of a color or a sound" (1970, p. 64). Why is it so difficult? The reason is clear enough: "We are anxiety-ridden animals. Our minds are continually active, fabricating an anxious, usually self-preoccupied *veil* which partially conceals the world" (p. 82). We are also *narrating* animals. By all indications, this is part of the problem too. Narrative anxiety "infects every aspect of life," according to Sartwell.

> For while the disciplinary matrix inscribes us, it also makes us anxious: anxious to please it, anxious to allow ourselves to be inscribed, anxious that we have not been thoroughly enough inscribed, anxious that our inscriptions have not been recently-enough updated, anxious that some present moment is not being turned to account, anxious that we are failing in our rationality, anxious that we are not perfect instruments, anxious that we are not perfect masters of instruments, anxious at our indifference, anxious at our ecstasy, anxious of being found out, anxious of finding ourselves out, anxious of incoherence, anxious about the future of projects, anxious about living in the present, anxious about the sacred. (2000, p. 66)

Sartwell goes on to acknowledge that "The lack of narrative is a kind of madness"—or at least can be. "(B)ut too much narrative is also a kind of madness" (p. 67). With this madness in mind, Sartwell moves in a similar direction to Murdoch:

> The deepest human needs and their satisfactions . . . take the form precisely of a letting-go, or a languorous lapse into silence. We take pleasure in eating a good meal, but not because it leads us toward salvation, or even because it leads us toward happiness considered as a property of a

whole life, but because it calls us into a present enjoyment wherein the imaginative reconstruction of the temporal flow is suspended. (p. 67)

Letting go brings one beyond narrative, or least that dimension of it that is tied to the autobiographical self. Does moving beyond narrative, as it is operative in the autobiographical self, facilitate the process of letting go? Or, to put the question somewhat differently: Does moving beyond the autobiographical self facilitate the deepening of the core self?

It is possible that the challenge of achieving the state about which Murdoch and Sartwell speak is made easier in dementia: With the removal, or at least the diminution, of the "self-preoccupied veil" that conceals the world, perhaps the world can more readily be *un*concealed (see Heidegger, 1971). Perhaps it is even possible that the ontological/spiritual identity I spoke about earlier and that Damasio seems to be considering in his idea of a core self may be further realized in this condition. Perhaps, that is, there is some sort of opening into the "beyond"—the world beyond narrative—that can allow this to occur. Murdoch speaks in this context of the "spiritual role" of music, for instance, and how art, more generally, "pierces the veil and gives sense to the notion of a reality which lies beyond appearance" (p. 86). She also speaks of the connection between such experience and mystical experience.

Let me be clear about this. I certainly do not wish to *equate* the later experience of dementia with mystical experience. This would be to romanticize dementia and to pathologize mysticism. Nevertheless, it may be that each, in their quite different ways of moving beyond narrative, offers a kind of deliverance, a reprieve from the anxiety and pressure of the autobiographical self. Whether this process of autobiographical unselfing has the redemptive outcome we are hoping for, only time will tell. For now, we have to work together to find resources, internal as well as external, to help my mother through some difficult days. Eating good meals together, as we often do, will undoubtedly help the process along.

REFERENCES

Bataille, G. (1988). *Inner experience.* Albany, NY: SUNY Press.

Damasio, A. (1999). *The feeling of what happens: Body and emotion in the making of consciousness.* San Diego, CA: Harcourt, Inc.

Freeman, M. (2000). When the story's over: Narrative foreclosure and the possibility of self-renewal. In M. Andrews, S. D. Sclater, C. Squire, & A. Treacher (Eds.), *Lines of narrative: Psychosocial perspectives,* 81–91. London: Routledge.

Freeman, M. (2002). Charting the narrative unconscious: Cultural memory and the challenge of autobiography. *Narrative Inquiry, 12,* 193–211.

Freeman, M. (2004). The priority of the Other: Mysticism's challenge to the legacy of the self. In J. Belzen & A. Geels (Eds.), *Mysticism: A variety of psychological approaches,* 213–234. Amsterdam: Rodopi.

Freeman, M. (2006). Autobiographische Erinnerung und das narrative Unbewusste In H. Welzer & H. J. Markowitsch (Eds.), *Warum Menschen sich erinnern können,* 129–143. Stuttgart, Germany: Klett-Cotta.

Heidegger, M. (1971). *Poetry, language, thought.* New York: Harper Colophon.
Murdoch, I. (1970). *The sovereignty of good.* London: Routledge.
Sartwell, C. (2000). *End of story: Toward an annihilation of language and history.* New York: SUNY.

Contributors

Jens Brockmeier is a Senior Scientist in the Department of Psychology of the Free University of Berlin and a Visiting Professor in the Department of Psychology of the University of Manitoba. His research is concerned with the cultural fabric of mind and language, with a focus on narrative as psychological, linguistic, and cultural form—issues he has explored both as empirical phenomena (in various languages and sociocultural contexts, as well as under conditions of illness and health), and as philosophical questions.

Pia Bülow is Assistant Professor in Communication in the Department of Health and Society at the University of Linköping, Sweden. She has published numerous papers on narrative and social interaction, especially focusing on illness narratives in institutional settings.

Georg Drakos, PhD, is Associate Professor in Ethnology at Stockholm University, Sweden. In his latest book, *Narratives in the World of Illness: Living with HIV/AIDS as a Relative in Sweden and Greece* (in Swedish, 2005), he extends and refines some of the argumentation in his doctoral thesis, *Empowering Body and Health: Leprosy and Self-understanding in Late Twentieth Century Greece* (in Swedish, 1997). Drakos has long been a driving force in a Nordic-Greek collaborative effort comprising several scholars in the humanities, social sciences, and medicine.

Arthur W. Frank is Professor of Sociology at the University of Calgary, Canada, and a pioneer of the study of illness narratives and its ethical implications. He is the author of a memoir of his own illness experiences, *At the Will of the Body* (1991; new edition, 2002), *The Wounded Storyteller* (1995), and most recently, *The Renewal of Generosity: Illness, Medicine, and How to Live* (2005).

Mark Freeman is Professor of Psychology at the College of the Holy Cross in Worcester, Massachusetts, USA. A leading figure in the steadily growing field of narrative psychology, he has written extensively on autobiography, self, and the narrative construction of identity. Among his books are *Finding the Muse* (1993) and *Rewriting the Self* (1993).

Lars-Christer Hydén is Professor of Health Communication at Linköping University, Sweden. His main focus is on language and social interaction in especially health settings. He has published extensively on illness and narrative. His main focus is on the role of narrative in the cultural interplay of illness and health. Ongoing research is concerned with narration in Alzheimer's disease and aphasia. He has previously, together with Sonja Olin Lauritzen, edited the book *Medical Technologies and the Life World: The Social Construction of Normality* (Routledge, 2006).

Margareta Hydén, PhD, is Professor of Social Work at Linköping University, Sweden, and a licenced psychotherapist. One of her books is *Woman Battering as a Marital Act: The Construction of a Violent Marriage* (1992). In her research she is concerned with narrative in contexts of family. An international expert on violence toward women, she recently has also worked with children who have witnessed domestic violence.

Cheryl F. Mattingly is Professor of Anthropology at University of Southern California, California, USA. She has written extensively about medical anthropology, psychological anthropology, narrative, phenomenology of illness and healing, and the culture of biomedicine, race and health. Her books include *Clinical Reasoning* (1994), *Healing Dramas and Clinical Plots* (1998), and *Narrative and the Cultural Construction of Illness and Healing* (2000).

Maria I. Medved is an Assistant Professor in the Department of Psychology at the University of Manitoba, Canada, and a licensed practicing psychologist. Her research is concerned with the way people deal with threats to their sense of self and identity in disease or after injury. She is especially interested in the narratives people tell themselves and others in order to cope with illness and disability and one main topic in this regard have been neurotrauma narratives.

Index